THE
FAMILY DOCTOR'S
HEALTH TIPS

by Keith W. Sehnert, M.D.

Meadowbrook Press
18318 Minnetonka Boulevard
Deephaven, Minnesota 55391

First printing October, 1981

Printed in the United States of America

ISBN (paperback): 0–915658–39–9
ISBN (hardcover): 0–915658–45–3

Library of Congress Cataloging in Publication Data

Sehnert, Keith W.
    The family doctor's health tips.
    Includes index.
    1. Health.   2. Medicine, Popular.   I. Title.
RA776.S452   613   81-16858
ISBN 0-915658-45-3   AACR2
ISBN 0-915658-39-9 (pbk.)

Art Direction and Design: Terry Dugan
Assistant Art Director: Sandra Falls
Illustrator: Shari Hohl and Associates
Production Manager: John Ware
Managing Editor: Kathe Grooms
Editor: Amy Rood

CONTENTS

SPECIAL FEATURES

Acknowledgments

I wish to thank Tim Rumsey, M.D., medical director, and Aleda Mathiowetz, R.N., health educator, medical self-care advocates from the Helping Hand Clinic in St. Paul, Minnesota; and Milton H. Seifert, Jr., M.D., family doctor and member of the "Patient Care" Management Medicine Advisory Board from Excelsior, Minnesota, for their great help and useful advice in reviewing the manuscript of **The Family Doctor's Health Tips.** *I'd like to give a special tip of my hat to the excellent laypeople who reviewed it, too: Linda Dugan and Nancy Palesch. And finally, thanks to all the people at Meadowbrook Press whose contributions helped shape the form and scope of this book.*

Acknowledgment is also made to the American Medical Association's Committee on Exercise and Physical Fitness for permission to adapt their report, "Evaluation for Exercise Participation," which appeared in the Journal of the American Medical Association (Vol. 219: No. 7, 1972).

The material on pp. 33–35 was adapted and reprinted with permission from Recreation Canada, Fitness and Amateur Sport Branch, Ottawa, Ontario.

The material on pp. 41–44, and selected material in Chapters 2 and 3, was adapted and reprinted from **Stress/Unstress** *by Keith W. Sehnert, M.D., with permission of Augsburg Publishing House.*

Selected materials were adapted and reprinted with permission from **How to Be Your Own Doctor (Sometimes)** *by Keith W. Sehnert, M.D. with Howard Eisenberg. © 1975 by Keith W. Sehnert and Howard Eisenberg. Reprinted by permission of Grosset and Dunlap, Inc., Publishers, 51 Madison Ave., New York, New York.*

The material in "One Event—Three Responses" on p. 47 is based on the work of Dr. Maxie C. Maultsby of the University of Kentucky.

Chapter 1

The Healthy Lifestyle

Have you ever noticed, after a bout with a bad sore throat or a headache, how *great* good health really feels? You don't just feel okay—the way most people do, day to day—but instead, you experience a kind of euphoric well-being. It seems almost a shame to return to ordinary health after a taste of that kind of wellness!

This book can't guarantee you euphoric well-being, or even good health. What it does give you, however, are the facts and tips you need to take charge of your own health. To a greater extent than you probably thought possible, you can make your own good health happen. And when an illness or emergency develops, you'll be ready to respond effectively and calmly.

There's nothing faddish or quirky about the tips here. After years of practice as a family physician, I know only too well that the keys to living a healthy lifestyle and knowing how to treat the common ills are not sensational news! But these are the facts:

• **Your lifestyle does affect your health.** It's been shown time and again that the sum total of your living habits is directly tied to your health—it's no longer fair to blame everything on germs and genes.

• **Fat kills.** Obese people have shorter life expectancies than lean people, a fact which crucially concerns (or should concern) the 30% of men and 40% of women over 40 in America who are obese.

• **Overdoing it on fat, salt, caffeine and sugar will hurt you.** And since the average American eats 4 times as much fat, 40 times as much salt and caffeine, and 100 times as much sugar as the body needs, it's pretty likely you can improve *your* health by paying attention to your intake of these ingredients in your diet.

• **Exercise improves your health.** Among 17,000 Harvard graduates studied over the past 25 years, those who exercise regularly have half the number of heart attacks as those who are sedentary.

• **Stress, badly managed, costs you.** It costs your general well-being, your physical health, and it affects others as well. In dollars, stress has been estimated to cost approximately $10 billion to $20 billion a year including lost work days, slight injuries, hospitalization and early stress-related deaths.

• **More accidents occur at home than anywhere else,** so for sheer impact on your health, removing risks from your home environment can really pay off.

• **Knowing how to manage your own health will save you money.** Programs in Washington, D.C.; Dayton, Ohio; and Boise, Idaho to teach families medical self-care skills saved those families over $200 a year in medical service bills, not to mention the illnesses they prevented.

How can you develop the habits and lifestyle that will give you the best possible odds of a long, healthy life? By making a strong commitment to improve your health. The information and tips in this book can serve as your guide. Each chapter addresses a key area you should evaluate and pay attention to in your health picture:

• the food you eat
• your physical fitness
• the state of your mind—and spirit
• the relative safety of your surroundings
• the quality of your health care
• your own ability to get the most from the health-care professionals
• your ability to treat common illnesses, injuries and emergencies

All the information presented here is sound and practical, and it's designed to be easy for you to read, remember and refer to. If you follow the tips for managing your own health that you'll find here, I predict that you could easily save $500 a year on health-care costs for a family of four—by simply cutting down on your need for office calls. In the long run, of course, you'll save much more—your health—by being aware of all you can do to take increased responsibility for your well-being. Use the self-tests, lists, checklists, tables, charts, diagrams and illustrations here to check up on your health.

Medicine has moved beyond its concern with infectious diseases caused by germs and pathogens (pneumonia, tuberculosis, polio, meningitis, mumps, measles and various bacterial and viral ills). We have discovered that they can be controlled by washing hands, covering faces with masks, immunizing people, prescribing antibiotics and medications, and so on. The major concern now is all of our "manmade pathogens": the cigarettes, alcohol, cars, guns, highly processed foods, polluted air and water and other hazards that seem to be part of our modern, highly technological lifestyle. The facts aren't all in, of course, but the fundamental message is clear—the healthier your lifestyle, the less threatened you'll be.

The changes you make in your way of living based on the tips in the following pages should start you thinking *and acting* like you're in charge of your health. Because when you take that responsibility to heart, your health picture is bound to improve. So here's to your health!

Life Expectancy Self-Test

This test enables you to estimate your life expectancy. To take it, note your score for each item in the appropriate column (leave blanks when you don't know the answer or when the item doesn't apply to you). As you finish each chart, subtotal the columns to get that chart's total score (positive or negative). At the end of the test, follow the directions for figuring out your approximate life expectancy. *Note:* people under 25 or who have coronary heart disease, cancer, cirrhosis of the liver, emphysema or other similar established diseases won't be able to get valid results from this test.

Chart A: Lifestyle

	+	−
1. **Personality.** Exceptionally good-natured, easy-going (+3); average (0); extremely anxious, tense most of the time (−6).	_____	_____
2. **Activity levels.** Physically active employment, or sedentary job with well-planned exercise program (+12); sedentary with moderate, regular exercise (0); sedentary work, no exercise program (−12).	_____	_____
3. **Home life.** Unusually pleasant, better than average (+6); average (0); unusually tense, family strife common (−9).	_____	_____
4. **Job.** Above average satisfaction (+3); average (0); discontented (−6).	_____	_____
5. **Air pollution.** Substantial exposure (−9).	_____	_____
6. **Smoking.** Nonsmoker (+6); occasional smoker (0); moderate, regular smoker—20 cigarettes, 5 cigars or 5 pipefuls daily (−12); heavy smoker—40 or more cigarettes daily (−24); daily marijuana smoker (−24).	_____	_____
7. **Alcohol consumption.** None or seldom (+6); moderate with fewer than 2 beers or 8 oz. wine or 2 oz. whiskey or hard liquor daily (−6); heavy, with more than above (−24).	_____	_____
8. **Food consumption.** Drink skim or low-fat milk only (+3); eat much roughage (+3); heavy meat, eaten 3 times daily (−6); over 2 pats butter daily (−6); over 4 cups coffee/ tea/cola daily (−6); usually add salt at table (−6). Enter total.	_____	_____
9. **Auto driving.** Regularly less than 20,000 miles annually and always wear seat belt (+3); regularly less than 20,000 but belt not always worn (0); more than 20,000 (−12).	_____	_____
10. **Drug use.** Use of street drugs other than marijuana (−36).	_____	_____
Subtotals	_____	_____
Chart A Total (+ or −)	_____	_____

Chart B: Physical Condition

	+	−

1. **Weight.** "Ideal" weight at age 20 was _____.
   If current weight is more than 20 pounds
   over that, score (−6) for each 20 pounds.
   If same as age 20, or less gain than
   10 pounds (+3).

2. **Blood pressure.** Under 40 years, if above
   130/80 (−12); over 40 years, if above
   140/90 (−12).

3. **Cholesterol.** Under 40 years, if above 220
   (−6); over 40 years, if above 250 (−6).

4. **Heart murmur.** Not an "innocent" type
   (−24).

5. **Heart murmur with history of rheumatic
   fever.** (−48).

6. **Pneumonia.** If bacterial pneumonia more
   than three times in life (−6).

7. **Asthma.** (−6).

8. **Rectal polyps.** (−6).

9. **Diabetes.** Adult onset type (−18).

10. **Depressions.** Severe, frequent (−12).

11. **Regular* medical checkup.** Complete
    (+12); partial (+6).

12. **Regular* dental checkup.** (+3).

Subtotals _____ _____

Chart B Total (+ or −) _____ _____

*"Regular" refers to well people who have thorough medical exams at least as
frequently as this: for age 60 and up, every year; 50-59, every 2 years; 40-49,
every 3 years; 30-39, every 5 years; 25-29, as required for jobs, insurance, military,
college, etc. More frequent medical checkups are recommended by other authorities.
Dental exams: twice yearly.

Chart C: Family and Social History

	+	−

1. **Father.** If alive and over 70 years, for each
   5 years above 70 (+3); if alive and under
   70 or dead after age 70 (0); if dead of
   medical causes (not accident) before
   70 (−3).

2. **Mother.** If alive and over 78 years, for each
   5 years above 78 (+3); if alive and under
   78 or dead after age 78 (0); if dead of medical
   causes (not accident) before 78 (−3).

3. **Marital status.** If married (0); unmarried
   and over 40 (−6).

4. **Home location.** Farm or small town (+3);
   suburb (0); large city (−6).

Subtotals _____ _____

Chart C Total (+ or −) _____ _____

Chart D: For Women Only

	+	−
1. Family history of breast cancer in mother or sisters. (−6).	___	___
2. Monthly breast self-exam. (+6).	___	___
3. Yearly breast exam by physician. (+6).	___	___
4. Pap smear yearly. (+6).	___	___
Subtotals	___	___
Chart D Total (+ or −)	___	___

Calculations

	+	−
Total from Chart A	___	___
Total from Chart B	___	___
Total from Chart C	___	___
Total from Chart D	___	___
Chart Subtotals	___	___
Chart Total (sum of the two Chart Subtotals, positive or negative)	___	___
Life Expectancy Score (Chart Total divided by 12)	___	

ANALYSIS

If your Life Expectancy Score is greater than zero, you stand a good chance of living that many years longer than the U.S. norm of 78 (for women) or 70 (for men).

If your Life Expectancy Score is less than zero, you stand a good chance of dying that many years earlier than the U.S. norm would predict for you. However, by improving your personal health habits and lifestyle, you can "buy time" and increase your life expectancy. The tips and information in this book will give you a strong foundation for improving your likelihood of a long, healthy life. In short, it's never too late to change!

Chapter 2

Nutrition and Your Health

When I was in high school my football coach used to tell me, "You are what you eat." Today, with our recent discoveries about wellness and healthy lifestyles, that saying should be changed a bit, perhaps to "You are what you *eat and do.*"

We've all known that what people eat and do affect their health, but it took the work of researchers in California to determine the details. Dr. Lester Breslow, former dean of the U.C.L.A. School of Public Health, his colleague Nedra Belloc and other scientists surveyed 6,928 adults to determine the health practices of ordinary people. When the study was completed they discovered that the Seven Golden Rules contributed to healthy lives.

Studies on this subject since the original survey in 1964 show that people who do these things have a physical status up to 30 years younger than people who follow few or none of the practices.

The last three of the Seven Golden Rules involve food and eating habits. Clearly, you'll greatly increase your prospects for a healthy, long life by paying attention to them!

Nutrition: The Whys and Whats of Eating

Unfortunately, most people get far too much of their nutritional information from the mass media, which tend to highlight what's sensational and ignore what's basic in a quest for newsworthiness. As Dr. Victor Herbert, a respected nutritionist, points out, "What's true about nutrition is not sensational and what's sensational is not true."

On the one hand, self-styled nutritionists mix facts, anecdotes and misconceptions to promote products and books as panaceas for most of the ills of mankind. They promise simplistic solutions for those who use their supplements, digestives and vitamins.

On the other hand, respected scientists view such solutions as

---

Seven Golden Rules

1. Don't smoke cigarettes.
2. Don't use alcohol at all, or use it moderately.
3. Get regular vigorous work or exercise.
4. Sleep 7–8 hours a day regularly.
5. Maintain proper weight.
6. Eat a nutritious breakfast every day.
7. Don't eat between meals.

ranging from deceptive and misleading to downright fraudulent. Dr. Herbert notes, "The willingness of the media to promote nutrition cultism, as long as it is sensational, is compounded by the unwillingness of most scientific journals to publish facts which could arouse the ire of cultists and promoters."

If "sensational" seems to be selling more than "sensible," is there any hope for directing our attention to sound rules for good nutrition? What basic guidelines can we follow?

The basic guidelines

When you weed out the fads and the fly-by-night cultists, you end up with some basic, unsensational nutritional guidelines that are true today and will still be true tomorrow:

Be moderate in all things—especially in what you eat and in the vitamins/minerals you take.

Eat a variety of foods. Food fads end up shortchanging you in some way.

Eat less salt and sugar.

Eat less fat and cholesterol.

Eat more foods with adequate fiber.

To lose weight, eat fewer calories each day than you burn up. Most people gain weight *not* because they eat too much, but because they *exercise too little.*

To gain weight, eat more than you burn up.

Drink plenty of water.

Common Misconceptions about Nutrition

These statements are all illustrations of commonly held misconceptions about nutrition.

- "More is better when it comes to vitamins."
- "Nutritional supplements are a quick, simple fix for many health problems."
- "The establishment (that is, the AMA and governmental agencies) is part of a conspiracy against healthy foods."
- "Doctors don't know anything about nutrition."
- "You can make up for all kinds of bad habits by taking the right amounts of the proper vitamins."

Common Questions and Answers about Food and Nutrition

 Are organic foods better than nonorganic?

A: No. Organic foods are more expensive, offer less variety and are *not* free from all toxic materials. (Pollutants consumed by animals are excreted in the manure used as organic fertilizers and are then absorbed from the soil into the "organic" plant.)

(continued)

Common Questions and Answers
about Food and Nutrition *(continued)*

Q: Should all breakfast cereals be avoided?

A: No. Enriched cereals are a good source of vitamins, especially if they are eaten with fruit and milk. Some cereals should be avoided if they contain large amounts of sugar. (Check the side panel of the box. If sugar, corn syrup or words that end in -ose—like *dextrose*—are the first or second ingredients, pick another type.)

Q: Are there any healthy snacks?

A: Yes, but eating between meals isn't good for you because it throws your metabolism off-balance. If you must snack occasionally, choose raisins, nuts, grapes or carrots rather than candy, cookies or cake.

Q: Are food additives okay?

A: Yes and no. Most food *preservatives,* by protecting you from spoiled food, are helpful; without them your choice of food would be severely limited. (Smoking, salting, sugar-curing, drying and pickling have been used for centuries to preserve food and keep it edible longer.) Some food *additives* (coloring and flavorings, for example) have been considered unsafe and have been withdrawn from use, but most others in use are okay. By "okay" I mean that they help some and probably don't hurt you.

Q: How much of your daily caloric intake goes for basic body maintenance, and how much goes for energy to go about your activities?

A: Assuming normal health and average caloric intake, as much as two-thirds of the calories an adult consumes each day are burned up just to keep the body temperature normal. The other third is burned up by exercise and other activities.

The Basic Four—A
New American Eating Guide

	Anytime	In Moderation	Now & Then
group 1 **Beans, Grains & Nuts** FOUR OR MORE SERVINGS/DAY	bread & rolls (whole grain) bulghur dried beans & peas (legumes) lentils oatmeal pasta, whole wheat rice, brown rye bread sprouts whole grain hot & cold cereals whole wheat matzoh	cornbread flour tortilla granola cereals hominy grits macaroni and cheese matzoh nuts pasta, except whole wheat peanut butter pizza refined, unsweetened cereals refried beans, commercial, or homemade in oil seeds soybeans tofu waffles or pancakes with syrup white bread & rolls white rice	croissant doughnut (yeast-leavened) presweetened breakfast cereals sticky buns stuffing (made with butter)
group 2 **Fruits & Vegetables** FOUR OR MORE SERVINGS/DAY	all fruits & vegetables, except those listed at right applesauce (unsweetened) unsweetened fruit juices unsalted vegetable juices potatoes, white or sweet	avocado cole slaw cranberry sauce (canned) dried fruit french fries, homemade in vegetable oil, commercial fried eggplant (vegetable oil) fruits canned in syrup gazpacho glazed carrots guacamole potatoes au gratin salted vegetable juices sweetened fruit juices vegetables canned with salt	coconut pickles
group 3 **Milk Products** CHILDREN: 3 TO 4/ADULTS: 2 SERVINGS/DAY	buttermilk made from skim milk lassi (low-fat yogurt & fruit juice drink) low-fat cottage cheese low-fat milk, 1% milkfat low-fat yogurt non-fat dry milk skim milk cheeses skim milk skim milk & banana shake	cocoa made with skim milk cottage cheese, regular, 4% milkfat frozen lowfat yogurt ice milk low-fat milk, 2% milkfat low-fat yogurt, sweetened mozzarella cheese, part-skim type only	cheesecake cheese fondue cheese souffle eggnog hard cheeses: bleu, brick, camembert, cheddar, muenster, swiss ice cream processed cheeses whole milk whole milk yogurt
group 4 **Poultry, Fish, Meat & Eggs** TWO SERVINGS/DAY VEGETARIANS: Nutrients in these foods can be obtained by eating more foods in Groups 1, 2 & 3	FISH cod flounder gefilte fish haddock halibut perch pollock rockfish shellfish, except shrimp sole tuna, water-packed EGG PRODUCTS egg whites only POULTRY chicken or turkey boiled, baked or roasted (no skin)	FISH (drained well, if canned) fried fish herring mackerel, canned salmon, pink, canned sardines shrimp tuna, oil-packed POULTRY chicken liver, baked or broiled fried chicken, homemade in vegetable oil chicken or turkey, boiled, baked or roasted (with skin) RED MEATS (trimmed of all outside fat!) flank steak leg or loin of lamb pork shoulder or loin, lean round steak or ground round rump roast sirloin steak, lean veal	POULTRY fried chicken, commercially prepared EGG cheese omelet egg yolk or whole egg (about 3/week) RED MEATS bacon beef liver, fried bologna corned beef ground beef ham, trimmed well hot dogs liverwurst pig's feet salami sausage spareribs untrimmed red meats

Nutrition Content

The Basic Four—fruits/vegetables, grains, animal/vegetable proteins, and dairy products—meet the daily needs of your body. They contain the carbohydrates, proteins, fats, fiber, vitamins and minerals that keep your body functioning well.

Proteins

The word *protein* means *primary* or *first* in Greek. It signifies that protein is of primary importance to life.

• **Proteins are used to repair, rebuild and replace** cells in your body. When you eat no protein for a long time, your body tissues shrink away because they get no materials with which to rebuild your cells.

• **Proteins contain "building blocks"** called *amino acids,* some of which are synthesized (produced in the body) and others of which come directly from the foods you eat. In order to have a properly functioning, healthy body, a person needs to get all the amino acids in proper proportions.

• **Imbalances.** In some situations, people suffer from an imbalance of essential amino acids. Such an imbalance can be avoided by eating protein foods from a wide variety of sources. Animal and dairy products (meat, eggs, poultry, fish, milk and cheese) tend to be *complete* sources of protein, while vegetable sources (beans, peas, grains and nuts) can be *incomplete.* However, it is possible to overcome that problem by pairing up complementary proteins to "create" complete ones.

Carbohydrates

Carbohydrates are your main source of energy—and potentially the main source of the body fat we collect.

• **When you digest foods,** carbohydrates are converted into blood sugar *(glucose).* Glucose is essential for muscular activity, nervous-system functions and body-temperature maintenance.

• **When you eat more carbohydrates than you need,** they are stored as *glycogen* in your liver and muscles. Once these "storehouses" are filled, any further excess is stored as body fat.

• **When you exercise,** glucose levels in your blood drop; first the glycogen and then the fat is converted to glucose to keep you supplied with energy.

Fats

Fats, like carbohydrates, are primary energy sources. Some fats also contain significant quantities of vitamins and essential fatty acids. Fats make food tastier, make up part of the structure of our cells and cushion our vital organs with fat pads that act as "shock absorbers" and have other important functions, as you'll see below.

• **Saturated fats:** butter, lard, chicken fat, coconut oil and hardened (hydrogenated) vegetable oils. Biochemists chose that term—*hydrogen*ated— because saturated fat molecules are "filled with hydrogen."

These fats are sources of energy and are carriers of fat-soluble vitamins.

• **Polyunsaturated fats:** liquid vegetable oils such as corn, soybean and sunflower. They supply *essential fatty acids,* the simple fats we need for manufacturing hormones, nerve cells, nerve coverings and other vital tissues. Examples are linoleic, linolenic and arachidonic acid.

• **Monounsaturated fats:** peanut and olive oils. These fats contain some hydrogen atoms and thus are partially saturated; they function much as do the polyunsaturated fats.

• **Cholesterol:** some of this material comes from the food you eat and some is actually manufactured in your body. In foods, it's a wax-like material present in fatty meats and dairy products; and although we often think of cholesterol as "bad," it has many good uses: it makes food tastier, aids in digestion and is used in the manufacture of some hormones and bile. When you consume large amounts of cholesterol, the manufacturing process slows down. Excessive intake leads to increased levels in the blood and deposits of the wax-like material in the veins and heart. Thus nutritionists recommend diets low in cholesterol (see p. 19).

Fiber

Fiber is what provides plants with their supporting structures: stems, pulp and skins.

• **Dietary fiber** serves as a natural laxative and thus prevents constipation.

• **Fiber, heart disease and cancer.** According to recent large-scale studies, primitive tribes of people in Africa who eat high-fiber foods have very little heart disease and colon cancer. It is only when they become "civilized" and eat the white man's "purified and refined" food that they get many of our modern ills. Fiber also tends to bind cholesterol and fats and keeps the blood level of cholesterol lower.

Vitamins

A vitamin is neither carbohydrate, fat or protein. It is an organic compound necessary for human metabolism.

• **Getting enough vitamins?** A balanced diet will supply you with all the vitamins you normally need.

• **Deficiencies.** Since vitamins are not made by the body in adequate amounts to sustain normal needs, deficiencies may produce conditions such as beriberi, scurvy, rickets or pellagra. Supplementary vitamins can correct such deficiencies.

Vitamin types

There are 13 substances that we call vitamins; they are classified as either *fat soluble* or *water soluble.*

• **Fat-soluble vitamins** (A, D, E and K) are stored in your body's fat. They function as regulators of metabolic activity. Because they can "pile up," you can overdose yourself with them and suffer serious consequences.

(continued on p. 14)

What Vitamins Do for You

Fat-Soluble Vitamins

Vitamin A
- **Use:** necessary for new cell growth and healthy tissues and essential for vision in dim light.
- **Deficiency:** causes night blindness, various eye maladies and rough, dry skin.
- **Excess:** in children and young people, causes increased pressure inside the skull that mimics brain tumors. Excesses in carotene, a vegetable form of A, can cause yellowing of skin.

Vitamin D
- **Use:** aids in the absorption of calcium and phosphorus in bone formation. Can be made in the body on exposure of the skin to sunlight.
- **Deficiency:** causes rickets (bowed legs, deformed spine and other bone deformation).
- **Excess:** causes nausea, weight loss, weakness, excessive urination and serious problems related to calcification of tissues and vital organs.

Vitamin E
- **Use:** acts as an antioxidant that helps prevent oxygen from destroying other substances in our diet. Many unsubstantiated claims are made for the value of E.
- **Deficiency:** causes a rare form of anemia in premature infants, but no clinical effects are associated with it in adults.
- **Excess:** self-medication with E in the hope that it will alleviate other conditions may cause problems.

Vitamin K
- **Use:** required for normal clotting of the blood. Comes in two natural forms: K_1, occurring in plants, and K_2, formed by bacteria in the intestinal tract. Also

(continued)

What Vitamins Do *(continued)*

comes as synthetic K, menadione.

- **Deficiency:** can cause bleeding disorders, hemorrhage and liver injury.

- **Excess:** can lead to harm, so synthetic K is dispensed only through prescription.

Water-Soluble Vitamins

Vitamin C

- **Use:** promotes growth and repair of tissue and the healing of wounds, aids in tooth and bone formation, and helps form collagen, a protein that holds tissues together.

- **Deficiency:** causes scurvy with symptoms of weakness, irritability, loss of weight, bleeding gums and easy bruising.

- **Excess:** may produce "rebound scurvy" in newborn infants of mothers taking large doses, adverse effects on growing bones, a false positive Clinitest for sugar and false negative Testape reports, renal problems, diarrhea, menstrual bleeding in pregnant women, destruction of B_{12} in food and other abnormalities.

B-Complex Vitamins

- **Vitamins:** B_1 (thiamine), B_2 (riboflavin), niacin, pantothenic acid, folic acid (folacin), B_6 (pyridoxine), B_{12} (cyancobalamin) and biotin.

- **Use:** important for energy and nervous functions, including your ability to handle stress.

- **Deficiency:** can cause beri-beri (B_1), pellagra (niacin), pernicious anemia (B_{12}) and other metabolic disorders with a wide variety of symptoms.

- **Excess:** may be hazardous despite claims from proponents of large doses of vitamins.

• **Water-soluble vitamins** (C and the eight B-vitamins) are not storeable and thus are eliminated as wastes when they are taken in excessive amounts. They function as coenzymes at the cell level of tissues. This means that they become a part of the cell and help regulate its chemical reactions.

Megavitamin therapy

• **Sensational and unsound,** megavitamin therapy is treatment with one or more vitamins in amounts *ten or more times* the Recommended Daily Allowances of the Committee on Dietary Allowances, Food and Nutrition Board, National Research Council of the United States. It is based on the simplistic assumption that more is better—which is not the case with vitamins! You can do real damage by overdoing it with them.

• **For more details,** write for the book, *Recommended Dietary Allowances,* Printing and Publishing Office, National Academy of Sciences, 2101 Constitution Avenue, Washington, D.C. 20418. The cost is $6.00.

Minerals

Today's consumers are increasingly aware of the importance of minerals in their diets. More than 60 inorganic elements have been found to be components in living organisms. Many are essential for human nutrition. Depending on how much of them you need, they are classi-

fied as *bulk* or *trace* minerals.

• **Bulk minerals.** You need such minerals as calcium, phosphorus, sulfur, magnesium, potassium, sodium and chloride in relatively large amounts (100 milligrams or more each day) for good health.

• **Trace minerals.** You only need these minerals in small amounts. They are iron, manganese, copper, iodine, zinc, cobalt, fluorine, selenium and a few others.

What minerals do

• **Body-building.** They support the building functions of the skeleton and all soft tissues.

• **Regulation.** They help regulate heartbeat, blood clotting, nerve responses, transportation of oxygen from the lungs to the tissues and maintenance of the internal pressure of body fluids.

Sources of minerals

• **Your regular diet.** If you eat a mixed diet of well-chosen foods that include the recommended amounts of animal and vegetable protein, you'll get most of the known minerals and trace minerals you need for good health, without taking a daily vitamin supplement.

• **Exceptions.** *Fluorine* (naturally present in some water supplies, absent in others) and *iodine* are exceptions; diets may need to be supplemented with these minerals. Women of child-bearing age may also need iron supplements.

• **Overdosing.** Sodium chloride—table salt—is a tasty and innocent-looking mineral that can be as dangerous as it is delightful. Most Americans eat far too much of it. A daily intake of one to two grams (one teaspoon) is needed for average temperature and work conditions. Excess salt can lead to high blood pressure, weight gain and problems of the heart and vascular system.

Our Changing Nutritional Habits

Changes in our lifestyles, our perceptions about food and the cost of eating are altering the way we eat. The *amount* of food that people eat—1,463 pounds a year, or over four pounds a day—has varied little over the past 20 years. However, the patterns of what people eat have shifted.

According to *U.S. News and World Report,* we have shifted toward eating more poultry, fish and meat; processed vegetables and fruits; fats, oils and sugars; cereal products; and cheese. And we are washing down almost 38 gallons (over 400 cans) of soft drinks per person each year. During the same 20 years, we've cut back on fresh vegetables and fruits; milk, cream and eggs; and coffee.

We have changed in the amount of time we spend eating out. Ten years ago we spent 29% of our food budgets in restaurants. Now we spend over 50% of our food dollars at fast-food places and restaurants, according to the American Dietetic Association. And a study by the restaurant-industry magazine, *Institutions,* reports that in 1980 the average household ate 6.4 of its 21 weekly meals out and spent $22.71 in the process.

Dietary goals

In 1977, the U.S. Senate's Select Committee on Nutrition and Human Needs, chaired by former Senator George McGovern, conducted exhaustive research on how Americans could improve their diet. The committee determined what proportions of fats, proteins and carbohydrates in average diets contribute to people's daily consumption, and established dietary goals —improved balances among those elements—which will ensure better health.

How do all the changes in our eating habits fit with the recommendations that were made during the Senate hearings?

• **On the good side,** we've increased consumption of poultry, fish and (more recently) complex carbohydrates.

• **On the bad side,** we're eating more sugar, sweeteners and soft drinks, but consuming fewer fresh vegetables and fruits.

What's Eaten More—and Less

	1979 (per person)	Change Since 1960		1979 (per person)	Change Since 1960
Soft drinks	37.5 gallons	Up 175.7%	Processed fruit	58.0 pounds	Up 15.3%
Poultry	61.6 pounds	Up 79.1%	Pork	65.0 pounds	Up 7.8%
Cheese	22.4 pounds	Up 71.0%	Flour, cereal products	150.0 pounds	Up 2.0%
Processed vegetables	65.0 pounds	Up 29.0%	Fresh vegetables	144.3 pounds	Down 1.2%
Fish	17.6 pounds	Up 28.5%	Fresh fruit	81.3 pounds	Down 9.7%
Fats, oils (including butter, margarine)	61.2 pounds	Up 26.2%	Milk, cream	32.9 gallons	Down 12.4%
Sugar, sweeteners	137.0 pounds	Up 26.2%	Eggs	274	Down 15.4%
Beef	79.6 pounds	Up 23.8%	Coffee	8.6 pounds	Down 25.9%

Dietary Goals Chart

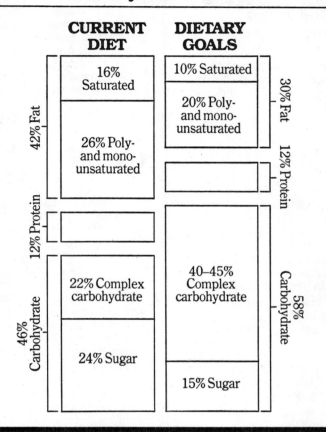

CURRENT DIET	DIETARY GOALS

Current Diet:
- 42% Fat
  - 16% Saturated
  - 26% Poly- and mono-unsaturated
- 12% Protein
- 46% Carbohydrate
  - 22% Complex carbohydrate
  - 24% Sugar

Dietary Goals:
- 30% Fat
  - 10% Saturated
  - 20% Poly- and mono-unsaturated
- 12% Protein
- 58% Carbohydrate
  - 40–45% Complex carbohydrate
  - 15% Sugar

Recommended Changes in Americans' Eating Habits

1. Decrease consumption of meat and increase consumption of poultry and fish.

2. Substitute low-fat milk for whole milk.

3. Decrease consumption of butter-fat, eggs, and other high cholesterol products.

4. Increase consumption of fruits, vegetables and whole grains.

5. Decrease consumption of foods high in fat and partially substitute polyunsaturated for saturated fat.

6. Decrease consumption of sugar and foods high in sugar content.

7. Decrease consumption of salt and foods high in salt content.

Source: Select Committee on Nutrition and Human Needs, United States Senate, U.S. Government Printing Office, Washington, D.C. 20418 (1977).

Eight Planning Tips for Nutritious Eating Habits

Here are some good general guidelines and several specific planning tips you can use to improve the quality and type of food you and your family eat.

1. Eat varied and balanced meals: select a variety of foods from the Basic Four. Not all foods contain all of the many nutrients, so protect yourself with many types of protein, carbohydrates, fats, vitamins and minerals.

2. Eat your food as near to its natural form as possible: choose a baked potato from your garden over dehydrated potatoes from the supermarket.

3. Eat less fat: select fewer high-fat meats, such as beef and pork, and use more fish and poultry. Consume more polyunsaturated fats (vegetable oils) than saturated fats (butter). Drink skim milk.

4. Eat less salt: take the salt shaker off the table! Add only half the salt called for in recipes. Cut down on foods with visible salt such as pretzels, potato chips and crackers. Use lemon juice and herbs as flavorings instead of salt.

5. Eat less sugar, to reduce the amount of sugar you eat, cut down on cookies, cakes and candies. Such foods are described by nutritionists as being "empty calories"—that is, carbohydrates with no protein, fat, vitamins or minerals. In addition, sugar, especially in sticky products, promotes tooth decay.

6. Eat more fruits, vegetables and whole grains: these foods are good sources of vitamins and minerals. They also have a high-fiber content that is beneficial in reducing the risk of intestinal disease.

7. Read the ingredient labels of all your food products: remember the label rule, "First is most." If your brand of margarine lists hydrogenated oil first, it will increase your blood level of cholesterol more than one that is made from less saturated fats like corn or sunflower oils.

8. Think twice about vitamin supplements: well-balanced meals provide enough vitamins and minerals for most people. The vitamin-mineral supplements taken for "nutritional insurance" may occasionally be helpful but are probably unnecessary.

How to cut down on sugar

There seems to be little doubt that the per-capita consumption of cane and beet sugars and of corn sweeteners has increased over the years. In 1920 it was 99 pounds a year; the amount in 1979 was up to 137 pounds. Dr. Ira Shannon, a professor of biochemistry, has noted that in the 1920s about 75% of our intake came from a grocery store in a bag marked *sugar.* "Now the pattern is completely reversed. We have lost our discretionary control over sugar because it is hidden."

Increases in tooth decay, obesity, diabetes and cardiovascular disease seem to be linked to increases in the amount of sugars in our diet. The problem can be identified; the solution is difficult but obvious: CUT DOWN ON SWEETS.

• **Program children** to reject sugary cereals and snacks, offering fruits, raw vegetables and unsweetened cereals exclusively. They'll get their sugars away from home anyway.

• **Drink water and fruit juices** with no added sugars—moderately—and save artificially sweetened gums and soft drinks as special treats.

• **Stop snacking.** Since sweets are so often tied to snack foods, cutting out between-meal eating will reduce sugar consumption too.

• **Don't be fooled:** sugar, glucose, dextrose, corn syrup, fructose, honey, molasses, maltose, invert sugar—all sugars give the same result. So read labels wisely.

How to cut down on fats and cholesterol

• **Eat smart.** Use more fish, chicken, turkey and veal for your meat courses.

• **Reduce your use of fatty meats.** Use less beef, lamb, pork and ham. Limit use of fatty "luncheon" and "variety" meats such as sausages, salami, frankfurters and liverwurst.

• **Instead of butter** and other solid cooking fats, use liquid vegetable oils and margarines high in polyunsaturated fats such as safflower oil.

• **Choose lean cuts of meat.** Trim visible fat, broil rather than pan-fry, and discard the fat that cooks out of the meat.

• **Instead of whole milk** and cheeses, use skimmed milk, skimmed-milk cheeses, low-fat cottage cheese and yogurt.

• **Eat more vegetables and fruit** rather than meat.

• **Prepare meatless meals** such as spaghetti with meatless sauce, meatless chili and vegetable soup.

• **Cut down on eggs.** Eat no more than three per week.

• **Get in the habit of saying no** to cream soups, fried foods, casseroles and other mixed dishes, creamed foods, gravies, ice creams, cakes, pies and creamy puddings.

How to shake the salt habit

• **Avoid visible salt**—on pretzels, chips, crackers, margaritas.

• **Don't add any at the table.** Grab for the pepper if you get the "shakes"!

• **Don't add salt when you cook.** See if you can please your palate (and your family's) without it first.

• **Use salt substitutes** if you really hanker for the taste. (Sea salt is *salt*. Try non-prescription ones like co-salt—available at pharmacies—if you want to give this tip a try.)

• **Get salt-conscious.** Learn to shop for and order foods that aren't loaded with salt.

Substitute Salt Products

You may want to cut down on your salt intake, but you still have an insatiable craving for the *taste* of salt. What can you do? Consider trying these substitute salt products. You can buy the following products from drug stores:

> Co-salt (Norcliff-Thayer)
> Neocurtasal (Winthrop)

These are available from grocery stores:

> Adolph's Salt Substitute
> Morton's Salt Substitute (blue package)
> Morton's Seasoned Salt Substitute (brown package)

Many customers seem to prefer Adolph's Salt Substitute over other products, but one caution for all products: *don't add the substitute during cooking*—it makes the food bitter.

Salty Wisdom

Here are some fascinating facts about salt—and its relationship to your health.

1. While millions of Americans today are literally and figuratively wading in salt up to their aortas, it was not always so. In the past (and still true in many parts of the world today), salt was a rarity and used only by the well-to-do.

2. The word *salary* comes from the Latin word *salarium,* or "salt money," originally paid to Roman soldiers.

3. When visitors come to the U.S. from Asia and central Africa, they often find the saltiness of our food so offensive that they can't eat it.

4. Most Americans eat 10 to 40 times the amount of salt they need each day. Much of their intake is concealed in commercially prepared foods—in grocery stores or at restaurants. A large fast-food hamburger with fries will put you over your daily quota.

5. Consumer groups and health professionals have recently been petitioning the Food and Drug Administration to move against salt in our processed food. A spokesman for one such group, the Center for Science in the Public Interest, noted that a 6-ounce can of Hunt's tomato paste contains 730 milligrams of salt, while the same can of Del Monte contains only 25 milligrams. Canned soups are also notorious for excess salt: one serving may contain a whole gram of salt—half of your day's limit!

6. It's this simple: *if you cut down on salt, your blood pressure may drop.* Subtracting salt can add new zip to your life by leaving you less fatigued.

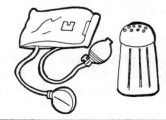

What Leads to Being Overweight?

1. Lack of activity. Most people are overweight not because they *eat too much* but because they *exercise too little.* Exercise, however, does more than burn calories. It is also important in the proper functioning of the appetite control center (the "appestat") in your brain. Low blood-sugar levels trigger hunger sensations much as low temperatures in your house, sensed by your thermostat, will turn on the furnace. Regular exercise and vigorous work help the appestat keep accurate. Little or no exercise can actually increase the appetite, according to studies!

2. Psychological conditioning. People who overeat were conditioned as children to associate food with comfort, consolation and reward. "If you are good, I'll give you a cookie." "Here, eat this and you'll feel better." "You got an A on your report card, so you deserve a big piece of pie." As these people grow up they look to food to provide emotional needs beyond its biological nutrients.

3. Heredity. If a child's parents are normal in weight, there is only a 7% chance of that child being overweight. If one parent is overweight, the child has a 40% chance of being overweight. If *both* parents are fat, the child has an 80% chance of being overweight! This is mainly due to family eating habits and in part to other metabolic factors, so you can see some modern wisdom in the old saying, "A bride inherits not only her mother's cookbook, but also her figure."

4. Childhood overfeeding. Recent studies show that overfeeding a child around the age of 12 months may increase the number of fat cells in the body by as much as 30%. This may lead to a lifetime of weight-control problems.

5. Glandular malfunction. Although many overweight people ascribe their problems to a "poor thyroid gland," few glands are actually to blame. (One wag has said the only "gland problems" are in the salivary gland — it is too active.) Carefully supervised thyroid supplements may be needed, however, by a few individuals.

Weight Control: Eating Less and Enjoying More

"I look at you, Mr. Shaw," said Alfred Hitchcock to the tall, lean and celebrated playwright, "and I know there is a famine in the land."

"I look at you, Mr. Hitchcock," replied George Bernard Shaw to the rotund film director-producer, "and I know who caused it."

The average American is overweight—women by 15 to 30 pounds, men by 20 to 30 pounds—and is becoming more so each year. Saying it simply, people get overweight because they take in more calories than they burn up.

In order to lose weight—and improve your health—you need to be aware of the causes of your weight problem. Then you can begin to do something to change the situation!

Formula for Ideal Weights

Sometimes the life insurance tables for figuring ideal weights are too complicated with bone size and so on. I prefer this simple formula:

Women: 100 + 5 pounds for each inch over 5 feet

Men: 106 + 6 pounds for each inch over 5 feet

If you exceed this rule by more than 10% to 20%, you are overweight. If you exceed it by more than 20%, you are obese.

Sensible and unsensible diets

Moderation and variety are the keys to any sensible diet. Any new book or plan that claims dietary "magic" should be viewed with suspicion, according to nutritional expert Dr. Victor Herbert. "They are nearly always a rip-off aimed at lining the author's pockets with book royalties."

Any sensible diet will take into account your need for exercise and sound nutrition. To help your diet work for you, here are some specific tips.

• **Make up your mind** that you really want to lose weight. If you don't, no diet will work.

• **Shop smartly.** What you don't buy you can't eat. Start this tactic at the supermarket or your neighborhood grocery store. Don't shop when you're hungry and buy less than you need: "less is better."

• **Harbor ill feelings about sugar.** It's the weight loser's worst enemy. Remember sugar, like a fugitive from prison, uses many aliases: "corn syrup," "invert sugar," "dextrose," "maltose," "sucrose" and so on.

• **Get more exercise.** If you don't, you're sunk to begin with. Plan vigorous exercise for 20 minutes three times each week.

• **Drink more water.** It is the only thing you can ingest with no calories. There are *lots* of calories in fresh fruit and vegetables.

• **Drink less alcohol.** Alcoholic spirits, including liquor, beer and wine, are loaded with calories.

• **Chew a lot.** Taste a lot. Smell a lot. Let your senses be used to guide the amount you eat. Chewing and savoring food takes time, and it's been found that people who are overweight are generally fast eaters.

• **Eat foods close to the source.** The closer you are to the source, the less chance of additives, processing and fattening alterations to your food.

• **Count the condiments.** Salad dressing, catsup, sauces and dips all add up fast.

• **Try not to eat alone.** Eating with others tends to make you converse and slows you down. Besides, it's more fun.

Nutrition resources

• Jane Brody, *Jane Brody's Nutrition Book* (W. W. Norton & Co., New York, 1981).

• Don Gerrard, *One Bowl* (Random House, New York, 1974).

• Victor Herbert, *Nutrition Cultism: Facts and Fictions* (George F. Stickney Co., Philadelphia, 1980).

• Bruce Lansky, *Successful Dieting Tips* (Meadowbrook Press, Deephaven, Minn., 1981).

Activity-Calorie Chart

(Based on the metabolism of a 150–pound person)

Activity	Calories/Min.	Time to Lose 1 lb.
Sleeping	1.3	44.9 hrs.
Sitting or reading	1.7	34.3 hrs.
Driving	2.0	29.2 hrs.
Light domestic work	3.0	19.4 hrs.
Bicycling or walking moderately	3.5	16.7 hrs.
Gardening	3.7	15.8 hrs.
Golf	4.2	13.9 hrs.
Bowling or lawn mowing (hand mower)	4.5	13.0 hrs.
Walking briskly or rowing	5.0	11.7 hrs.
Badminton or square dancing	5.8	10.0 hrs.
Tennis	7.0	8.3 hrs.
Skiing, squash or handball	10.0	5.8 hrs.
Bicycling briskly	11.0	5.3 hrs.
Running	15.0	3.9 hrs.

Nutritional Problems

There are many situations when persons are put on special
diets—diabetic, low salt, low cholesterol or whatever—by
their physician. There are nutritional patterns that may
be related to hyperactivity and hypoglycemia. There are also
many controversies about sugar and other substances in
our diet. What should one know? What are the problems?
What are the solutions?

Diabetes   A deficiency or absence of sugar-regulat-
                     ing insulin. In the U.S. about 5% of the
                     population has known diabetes, but perhaps
                     40% of all diabetes is undetected. The
                     vast majority (90%) of people with adult-
                     onset diabetes are overweight or obese.
                     In all forms of diabetes, disturbances in
                     metabolism of carbohydrates, fats and pro-
                     tein occur. Diabetes can be controlled by
                     limiting sugars and balancing calories with
                     regular physical activity, plus medications
                     and injections, if required. A program of
                     treatment and meal plans tailored to each
                     individual's condition and needs is worked
                     out by a physician or nutritionist.

Hypoglycemia   Low sugar levels in the blood (the oppo-
                     site of diabetes). Widespread media cover-
                     age of this condition has caused many
                     people to diagnose themselves with this
                     disorder. The danger is that its symptoms—
                     trembling, sweating, yawning, low energy
                     levels, headaches, fatigue—may match
                     those of other serious disorders of the liver,
                     pancreas, brain and other vital organs, not
                     to mention emotional problems. If you sus-
                     pect you are hypoglycemic or you have
                     a family history of diabetes, get a 6-hour
                     glucose tolerance test. Keep a record of
                     what and when you eat and how you
                     feel. A program of balanced nutrition,
                     suited to your particular condition and
                     developed for you by a professional nu-
                     tritionist, usually controls the symptoms.
                     (A low-carbohydrate, high-protein diet eaten

(continued)

Nutritional Problems *(continued)*

	in six small meals per day is often helpful.) You may also want to consider emotional counseling.
Hypertension	High blood pressure, which affects more than 23 million Americans. It contributes toward strokes, speeds arteriosclerosis (hardening of the arteries) and is a significant factor in the 650,000 heart attacks that occur each year. Salt is the culprit here: you should limit your intake to two grams (one teaspoonful) a day—in *all* your food—unless you are already under further restrictions.
High Blood (Serum) Cholesterol	Unnaturally high concentrations of fats dissolved in your blood tend to deposit in the walls of your arteries and reduce circulation. Deposits can contribute to strokes and heart attacks. There's some dispute over how severely most Americans need to control their fat intake; physicians and nutritionists agree that moderation in your cholesterol and saturated-fats consumption is a sound plan.
Hyperactivity	Increased motor activity in people of any age, but often seen in children. Some observers estimate that 5 million American children are hyperactive. The more than 3,000 food additives we have in our food is cited by Dr. Ben Feingold and others as a cause of hyperactivity. Other persons reject that view, but the facts seem to indicate that additives do have some adverse effects on some children. Regardless of whether restricting a child's intake of additives in itself cuts down on hyperactivity, or helps by increasing the interplay between parents and children who follow Feingold diets, the diets do seem to work for many people.

Chapter 3

The Many Roads to Fitness

You don't have to look very far to find evidence of a great current interest in America in taking better care of the body. In recent months I've seen the following news items.

• *Time* magazine is paying $400 of the $500 fee for all employees over 35 years of age who signed up for jogging exercise at New York's Cardio-Fitness Center.

• **Deseret Pharmaceuticals, Inc.** installed six exercise bicycles, strategically placed throughout the Sandy, Utah, headquarters for use by its 2,000 employees.

• **Officials at Pepsi Cola Corporation** completed arrangements for jogging tracks, courts for basketball, tennis and volleyball, a football field and a baseball diamond at their headquarters in Purchase, New York.

• **The Public Advocate's office** in San Francisco, a small poverty-law office, reported that their six lawyers and 25 clerks run each day.

Benefits of Exercise

What are the payoffs for the many Americans who are exercising? They are both physical and mental.

Physical benefits

Arthur S. Leon, M.D., an internationally recognized exercise psysiologist and health-sport expert at the University of Minnesota's Laboratory of Physiological Hygiene says exercise helps through:

• **getting more blood to the heart** to provide it oxygen and nourishment

• **improving the heart's ability to function** as a pump and the blood vessels' ability to carry blood to the rest of the body

• **slowing the heartbeat** and lowering blood pressure

• **making body muscles firmer** (and stronger)

• **lowering body weight** and the amount of fat in body tissue

• **lowering blood cholesterol** and other fats in the blood

• **improving the metabolism of sugar** (even for diabetics)

• **improving other health habits** (fit people tend to cut down on cigarettes, junk foods)

• **lowering tension** and other effects of stress

Mental benefits

In addition to all these physical benefits, there is evidence that exercise helps relieve depression. As Ronald M. Lawrence of UCLA and president of the American Medical Joggers' Association, an organization with over 3,000 members, says, "Man was meant to be a moving animal, but he's become sedentary. Distance running can bring us back to the basics of what we're here for."

One of the first documented studies on running was done by John Greist at the University of Wisconsin. Studies there in 1976 showed that jogging offered a better treatment for depression than psychotherapy.

• **Jogging had a better cure rate.** Six of eight clinically depressed patients were cured after a 10-week running program (an extraordinary 75% cure rate!). For another group of 28 depressed patients, 30–45 minutes of jogging three times a week was at least as effective as talk therapy.

• **Exercise beats pills.** Other psychiatrists have also found that exercise beats medication in controlling depression.

• **Running therapists,** like Thaddeus Kostrubala, a psychiatrist, marathoner and author of *The Joy of Running,* have started practicing psychotherapy while they jog alongside their patients. Jerome Katz of the Menninger Foundation says that jogging helps patients get talkative, but cautions, "The enthusiastic claims of instant cures of depression have to be evaluated with a great deal of salt."

• **The real secret,** according to one non-medical observer (Clinton Cox, of the *New York Daily News*), is that "It's almost impossible to worry about your job or other such mundane pursuits when your body is in total agony!"

Questions and Answers about Exercise

Q: Do salt tablets help you avoid fatigue when you exercise?

A: No. Unless you sweat enough to soak your clothes for an hour or two (as you would playing tennis or running on a hot day in late August), salt tablets can be worse than no salt at all. Salt attracts water and draws it from the tissues, *increasing* dehydration and the chance of fatigue. Tablets can also cause symptoms themselves as they lay on the mucous membrane lining of your stomach and produce enough irritation to actually make you nauseated. If you expect a vigorous workout, you would be better off to add some extra salt to your food—or to eat a handful of salted peanuts.

(continued)

Questions and Answers *(continued)*

Q: Should you put on a sweater or warm-up suit right after you finish vigorous exercise?

A: No. When you put on a sweater immediately after you exercise, you actually interfere with your body's normal attempts to get rid of heat. The sweater should be put on later when your sweating has subsided and you no longer feel hot.

Q: Should you drink water or other liquids immediately after (or even during) exercise?

A: Yes. Replace lost fluids immediately. Don't wait until you get thirsty. A good rule to follow is to drink an 8-oz. glass of water before you exercise, and then replace the fluids with water or juices when exercising, as you get dehydrated. A good rule to follow: one glass for every five miles of running.

Q: Can you get any good out of occasional exercise?

A: That depends on what "occasional" means, though occasional exercise is better than none. Most experts agree that if you get 20 minutes of vigorous aerobic exercise three times weekly (but *not* on consecutive days or only on weekends), you will receive cardiovascular benefits. But remember, the exercise should be vigorous. More haphazard exercise is decidedly less good for you.

Q: Does the over-fifty set have to stick to vigorous walking?

A: Absolutely not! Go to any YMCA, YWCA or athletic club and you'll find active senior citizens working out, running or swimming. Age alone is not a barrier to exercise. The literature on sports medicine and physical fitness is filled with examples of runners and swimmers who maintain vigorous exercise into their 80s and 90s. There is even the example of one man from California who ran regularly until he was 102!

Experts warn, however, that it is dangerous for sedentary persons older than 35 years to initiate *heavy* exercise. They are advised to have an evaluation by a knowledgeable doctor and then to start their exercise program slowly and build it gradually.

Beginning an Exercise Program

If you are one of the over 100 million American men or women who are in good general health but get little or no regular exercise, how should you start? Slowly! Even if your heart can take the stress, your joints, bones and muscles need time to adjust. Here's how you should "gear up" your body so that you can soon begin feeling better — and looking better.

Starting New Exercise Habits

1. **Get up a half hour early** and take a brisk walk, jog or bike for 15 minutes before breakfast.

2. **Use your feet** and rest your car. When you must drive to work or to the grocery store, park in the farthest corner of the lot; then walk to and from your car.

3. **On the way to work,** get off the bus or the train several blocks early and walk the rest of the way. At work, use the stairs instead of elevators.

4. **At noon,** "brown-bag it" and engage in some sort of exercise program for a half hour with the time saved.

5. **Take "exercise breaks"** — not "coffee breaks" — and walk briskly up and down the halls or stairs.

6. **After work,** instead of the two martinis before dinner, take two laps around the block.

When exercise is risky

If you are one of the 5% to 10% of the population who has a significant medical or health problem, what should you do? The American Medical Association's Committee on Exercise and Physical Fitness has said that there are some persons for whom *no exercise should be undertaken.* These are people who have the following medical conditions:

• **Active or recent myocarditis** (inflammation of the heart muscle)

• **Recent pulmonary embolism** (blood clot in the lung)

• **Congestive heart failure**

• **Arrythmia** from third degree A-V block (uneven heartbeat), or if using fixed-rate pacemakers

• **Aortic aneurysm** (ballooning of normal blood vessel wall to heart)

• **Ventricular aneurysm** (ballooning of normal heart wall)

• **Liver degeneration** (liver failure)

• **Congenital heart disease with cyanosis** (impaired circulation with bluish skin color)

When a check-up is recommended

The AMA committee also agreed that any person who has the following medical problems needs a medical history and extensive evaluation by a physician before an exercise program should be considered:

- **Acute or chronic infectious disease**
- **Diabetes** that is not well controlled
- **Marked obesity**
- **Psychosis** or severe neurosis
- **Central nervous system disease**
- **Musculo-skeletal disease** involving spine and lower extremities
- **Active liver disease**
- **Renal disease** with nitrogen retention (kidney failure)
- **Severe anemia** (iron deficiency in the blood)
- **Significant hypertension** (diastolic high blood pressure)
- **Angina pectoris** or other signs of myocardial insufficiency (chest pain on exertion)
- **Cardiomegaly** (malformation of the heart)
- **Arrythmia** from second degree A-V block, ventricular tachycardia or atrial fibrillation (irregular or abnormal fast heartbeats)
- **Significant disease of heart valves** or larger blood vessels
- **Congenital heart disease without cyanosis** (bluishness)
- **Phlebothrombosis** or thrombophlebitis (inflammation of veins)
- **Current use of drugs such as reserpine,** propranolol hydrochloride, guanethidine sulfate, guinidine sulfate, nitroglycerin (or other vascular dilators), procainamide hydrochloride, digitalis, catecholamines, ganglionic blocking agents, insulin or psychotropic drugs

What You Can Do Yourself

Assuming you're in basically good health, you should be able to develop your own conditioning program and, through it, improve your fitness. When you're in good condition, you can select a sport or activity for regular exercise.

Conditioning

Here is a collection of simple conditioning tips. They apply mainly to that most popular exercise of all, running, but are equally appropriate for all vigorous exercise programs.

- **Take the talk test.** You should be able to talk while you exercise. If you can't, you're working too hard—or running too fast—and should slow down.

- **Warm up and cool down.** Always do stretching and warm-up exercises before starting your activity. Do leg and back stretches, push-ups and sit-ups before you start. When you are ready to run, begin with a slow trot. Finish with a cool-down walk.

- **Don't be intimidated.** Do your own thing, at your own speed, in your own way.

- **Learn your body's capabilities.** If you are tight-jointed and stiff, you may need stretching or limbering calisthenics for several weeks before starting an exercise program.

Limbering and Warm-Up Exercises

Each time before you start any calisthenics or athletic activities, you should allow your body a chance to get ready for the additional demands you're about to place on it. Athletes know that injuries happen more often to people who haven't warmed up, and for that reason they bend and stretch before games and practices. You should too!

To limber the upper body
- Stand with legs astride, hands on hips.
- Rotate the upper body clockwise to the count of 100.
- Stop and then rotate in the opposite direction to the count of 100.

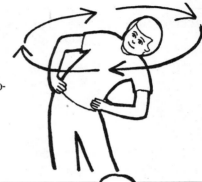

To stretch the hamstring muscle
(in the back of the leg)
- With left leg raised up on a counter or park bench, gently lean forward on that leg for the count of 30.
- Repeat, leaning on the right leg.

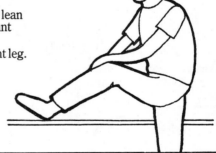

To stretch the achilles tendon
(heel cord)
- With feet parallel, stand back 18″ from a wall or tree.
- Place your hands on the surface and lean forward with knees and hips straight, until you feel the pull behind your knees. Hold for the count of 100. *Note:* ease up if this causes pain or distress.
- Stop, return to your upright position, and repeat the exercise as above once more before starting your other activities.

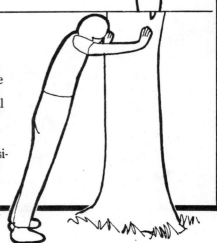

Know Your Kinds of Exercise

Isotonic	Rhythmic, repetitive exercise that involves motion. Improved blood circulation comes from the alternation between tensing and relaxing the muscles. Isotonic exercises can be either aerobic (calisthenics, horseshoe pitching, archery) or anaerobic (weight lifting).
Isometric	Exercise with very little movement, like pushing your hands against each other or lifting or pushing against an object that won't move. Although isometric exercises may develop muscle tone and can make you stronger, they don't improve your heart conditioning and may even be dangerous for heart patients. That is because they can cause the muscles involved to get shorter and tense up, squeezing blood vessels and decreasing the flow of blood through the heart.
Aerobic	Exercise that can be carried on for 15 or more minutes is generally aerobic. Aerobic exercise is steady, "non-stop" activity. Examples include swimming, jogging, cycling and walking.
Anaerobic	Exercise that is short in duration, "stop-and-go" in rhythm, and low intensity in effort. Examples include tennis and golf.

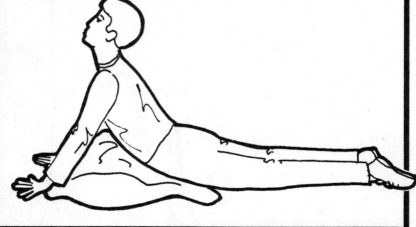

An Exercise Break

The aim of an exercise break is to stimulate circulation, improve posture, relax tense muscles and counteract boredom or mental fatigue. The aim is not to increase physical fitness, so it should not be strenuous enough to cause sweating, but if you do these vigorously, your condition will improve.

You should be able to do the complete cycle in 7 to 8 minutes. Doing the exercises to peppy music makes it actually fun!

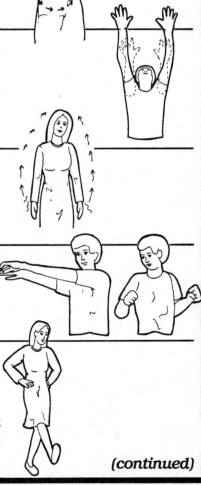

1. Shoulder Rolling

Stand relaxed. Raise one shoulder, slowly pull backward and then relax. Alternate with other shoulder. Make sure arms and hands are relaxed throughout. After eight rolls, repeat in reverse direction. Do four pairs of rolls.

2. Finger Exercise

Clench fists, arms bent; then stretch out all fingers with explosive movement, while stretching arms out overhead. Bend arms again and repeat. Vary arm positions from overhead to "Y" position, to side, etc. Do 12 to 16 times.

3. Wrist Loosening

Shake out hands from wrists, arms relaxed down. Continue shaking while lifting arms up to side and overhead, and then lowering back down. Repeat four to six times.

4. Swimming

Stretch arms out in front, pull back in wide circle to shoulders, as in the breast stroke, tightening up back muscles. Then stretch arms forward and repeat six to eight times.

5. Step-Kicks

Hop once on right foot, hop on right again while kicking up left foot across front. Hop onto left foot to side, then hop again kicking right foot across front. Repeat double hops on each foot; change kick part time to time (i.e., kick higher; kick to side, etc.). Keep kicking for about half a minute.

(continued)

An Exercise Break *(continued)*

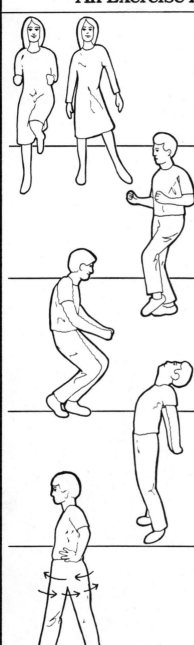

6. Knee-Lifts

Keeping rhythm by gentle bending of one knee, lift other knee up and across front, slapping knee with hands, and then stretch foot out to side. Do four knee lifts with one leg, then switch to four counts other leg. Complete four to six pairs of lifts.

7. Pedaling

Begin by gentle pedaling action, rolling up from heel to toe, alternating feet. Body is entirely relaxed. Build up to gentle jogging on the spot, lifting feet slightly off the ground, and continue for half a minute.

8. Knee Bends and Arm Swings

Put your feet apart; do a gentle knee bend and straighten up. Keep up a fast rhythm. Then add arm swings, any way, and continue for 20 to 30 seconds.

9. Back Exercise

Bend knees slightly; clasp hands behind back. Slowly pull shoulders and head back; arch upper back, keeping elbows straight. Hold; relax head and back, drooping shoulders forward. Repeat six to eight times.

10. Trunk Twists

Set feet apart, knees slightly bent, hands on hips. Twist to one side, gently, three times and face center on fourth count. Repeat to opposite side. Complete six to eight pairs of twists.

(continued)

An Exercise Break *(continued)*

11. Side Leans

(a) Stand with feet apart, arms relaxed at sides. Bounce *gently* to one side three times, reaching down the leg with hand. Straighten up on fourth count. Repeat to other side. Do four times on each side.

(b) *Add arms:* Reach up over head with left arm and lean to *right* three times and up. Repeat other side; do four times each side.

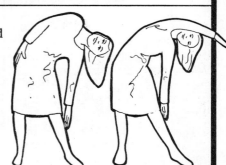

12. Neck Exercise

Stand straight, head to one side; slowly roll head down on chest and up to other side (two counts). Stretch head back and look at the floor over your shoulder (two counts). Repeat to other side. Do this four times on each side.

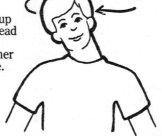

13. Arm Circles and Deep Breathing

Start with arms at sides, palms facing out. Slowly raise arms up in wide circle while breathing in deeply and slowly, finishing with arms stretched up overhead (four counts total). Reverse motion; breathe out slowly, while bringing arms down slowly with palms facing downward (four counts). Repeat four to six times.

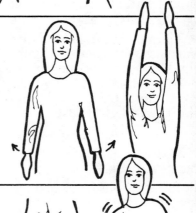

14. Shake-Out

General loosening of all joints — small kicking, shaking out from ankle, loose shaking of arms and wrists, shoulder shrugs, etc. (for about 15 seconds).

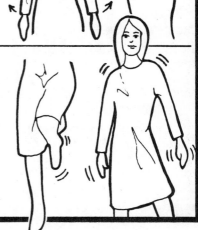

Aerobic exercise

Aerobic exercises — jogging, dancing, biking—allow you to get enough oxygen while you do them so that you can keep them up for more than 15 minutes. When you can do these exercises that long, you get real benefits for your heart's conditioning.

Because your pulse is needed as a guide to aerobic activity, you should learn to take your pulse at your wrist or on your neck at the angle of the jaw. Initially, you will not be exercising at a level to increase your heart rate enough to achieve changes in condition, but that will come with time.

• **With your hand held palm upward,** feel with the first two fingers (index and third) of the other hand at the outside of your wrist near base of your thumb.

• **Using a watch that measures seconds,** count the pulse for 30 seconds and multiply by two. The normal resting pulse for adults is 60 to 70. For children, it is slightly faster.

Finding your target pulse

In the early stages of training, use your target pulse to make sure you aren't exercising too vigorously. The following guidelines can be used:

• **If you are in poor condition,** take 150 and subtract your age. This is your maximum (or target) pulse while exercising.

• **If you are in fair to good condition,** take 170 and sub- tract your age. This is your maximum (or target) pulse while exercising.

Choosing a fitness activity

When you've completed your conditioning program, it's time to choose a sport or activity (or several) to do for fun and fitness. Whatever you choose should offer you ample opportunities to:

• **Move.** The benefit from walking, biking, hiking or jogging is that these activities burn up calories (see page 37).

• **Stretch and breathe deeply.** Deep breathing and stretching help you to relieve tension and to relax. These movements should be a part of any exercise you choose.

• **Bend, twist and swing.** Flexibility and agility are as important as muscular endurance and strength. Remember that flexibility refers to the range of movements of the joints.

• **Enjoy yourself.** When exercise is enjoyable, it's relaxing and gives physical, mental and social benefits.

• **Set your own pace.** Take three or four months of training to achieve your target pulse.

• **Do aerobic activity.** This type of exercise should be intense enough to increase your heart rate, make you perspire and breathe so rapidly you are not able to talk. After warming up, activity should be sustained for 15 minutes to provide aerobic conditioning effects.

Sports and Activities that Promote Fitness

Individual Activities	Group Activities	
Bicycling	Badminton	Judo
Calisthenics	Basketball	Karate
Chopping wood	Canoeing	Ping-pong
Hiking	Dancing	Racquetball
Horseback riding	Fencing	Soccer
Jogging	Football	Squash
Jumping rope	Golf (no carts allowed)	Tennis
Rowing	Handball	Water-skiing
Running	Jazzercise	Wrestling
Skating		
Skiing (cross-country)		
Skiing (downhill)		
Swimming		
Walking (briskly)		

What Are the Energy Requirements for Your Sport?

Activity	Calories Burned per Hour
Bicycling (5.5 m.p.h.)	210
Gardening	240
Golfing	250
Bowling	270
Playing tennis (doubles)	350
Walking (3.5 m.p.h.)	350
Playing ping-pong	350
Chopping wood	400
Playing tennis (singles)	450
Downhill skiing	450
Playing handball	550
Doing vigorous calisthenics	550
Dancing (fast)	600
Bicycling (13 m.p.h.)	660
Swimming	750
Running (10 m.p.h.)	900
Cross-country skiing	1,000

Fitness resources

•Kenneth H. Cooper, *The Aerobic Way* (Bantam Books, New York, 1977).

• James F. Fixx, *The Complete Book of Running* (Random House, New York, 1977).

Chapter 4

Your Mind and How to Understand It

Even little toddlers know there's a connection between body and mind: before they can talk, they can "read" their parents' physical signs of emotions, whether positive or negative. As they grow older they learn to read more subtle signs than the red faces of anger or the twinkling eyes of happiness; they grow adept at reading body language so they can sense anger even when a parent's back is turned, just by subconsciously noting the tension in the parent's shoulders.

Indeed, parents sometimes need to learn that very young children will pick up on emotions not aimed at them—anger at a boss or spouse, for instance —and assume they are the targets. Unless parents correct that misapprehension, children may shoulder a lot of blame and guilt that's not truly theirs.

So in practice we all know our minds and bodies are intimately connected. Yet our understanding of that connection is quite primitive, even though it's improving.

• **Ancient Greeks** thought that mental imbalances and moods were caused by excesses of body fluids, "humors," that somehow displaced the body's organs. Such excesses could lead to melancholy (literally, "black bile") or other extreme moods.

• **Colonial Americans** thought mental aberrations were caused by the devil, who had to be thrown out of the body, no matter what the cost to the possessed victim. Thus many "witches" were burned for their mental imbalances, creating in turn a form of mass hysteria that caused many more people to appear deranged.

• **Present-day researchers** are readdressing the mind-body connection in both its covert forms (high blood pressure resulting from stress) and its overt forms (loss of sleep due to lack of exercise, causing mental inefficiency). This chapter touches on some of the important issues in this area as they affect you.

Stress Management

You probably know someone like Bill Keller: his emotional "motor" has been tuned to "idle fast" all of his life. Bill is in business. After 20 years in that work, he's a success as vice-president of a firm and recognized expert in his special field. There is just one problem—he hasn't learned to *manage* the stress associated with his work and the only method he has

The Mind-Body Connection

We all tend to think that our emotions lead independent lives—that we don't really control them so much as they "happen" in response to external events. But as this diagram illustrates, emotional and physical responses occur at the end of a sequence of steps that we often can learn to shape consciously.

• Your sense organs (eyes, ears, nose, tastebuds, nerve endings) convey *perceptions,* the raw data from whatever happens in the world outside, to your brain.

• Your brain organizes that data and, as you think about the events, you *evaluate* them in a process that's very much like talking to yourself. In this process you assign a positive, neutral or negative value to the event you have perceived.

• Finally, your brain instructs your body to make its *response*: a different portion of the brain may experience an emotion, a part of your body may move, an organ or system in your body may develop a symptom of illness (an ulcer in response to tension).

Viewed in this way, you can see how stressful, negative emotions and even illnesses may be avoidable if you can teach yourself to evaluate as many events as possible in positive or neutral ways.

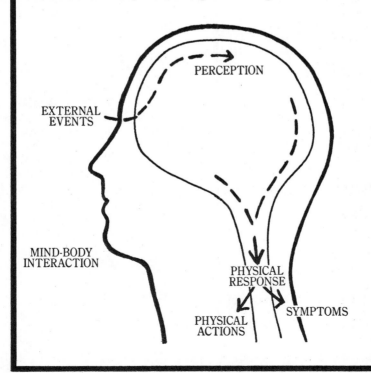

used to "control" his stress, alcohol, will destroy him unless he takes steps to change things soon.

You may also know a woman like Kari Olson. Her life spins about her in an almost uncontrolled manner, playing havoc with her and others. The surprising thing about Kari is that you'd think some of her professional training as a nurse would have given her some personal insight on stress, but, unfortunately, it hasn't. Kari finds herself approaching 30, divorced and — adding injury to insult — unable to work for the last three months because of a whiplash condition she obtained in a car accident.

On the surface there doesn't seem to be much in common between these two people. It is only when you look at their inability to slow down their emotional motors that you find common ground. If you were to ask them about their feelings after a busy or stressful day, both would describe how they felt with statements like these:

• "I was uptight all day."
• "I haven't been so irritable since I can't remember when."
• "I'm ready to blow up."
• "If that person says one more thing, I'll scream."
• "I haven't had a minute to breathe since I started work this morning."

Both Bill and Kari are threatening their physical well-being (not to mention the quality of their own lives as they live them, day in and day out), by not attending to their mental well-being. To be sure, both of them can identify the problem — they both notice a decline in the quality of their work and their job performance when they have had high levels of anxiety over several days. But they need to learn how to handle stress and anxiety — for their *own* good. Is it possible for people like these to understand and alter their stress-handling habits? Can they learn ways to help control their stress-laden lives before serious trouble develops?

Understanding your mind and emotions

These days, a great deal of attention is being paid to the effects of stress on people's minds and bodies. Before we plunge into that subject, however, I want to make two very important points.

• **First, stress is nonspecific,** in and of itself. It's the degree of stress you experience, paired with your ability to handle it, that gives it a positive or negative quality.

• **Second, you determine how stress affects you.** Your habits, abilities and experience in handling stress, more than the nature of the stress itself, are the primary determinants of its effects on you. Therefore, skill and practice in stress management lie at the root of your emotional and physical health.

Eustress and distress

Part of the ability to manage stress well comes from an informed sense of your own tolerance and need for it.

Test Your Own Stress Level

Evaluate your stress level by completing the test below, originally developed by Drs. T. H. Holmes and R. H. Rahe. Circle the scores of the events you have experienced in the last 12 months. Total your score and turn the page for an analysis.

Life event	Value
1. Death of a spouse	100
2. Divorce	73
3. Marital separation	65
4. Jail term	63
5. Death of a close family member	63
6. Personal injury or illness	53
7. Marriage	50
8. Fired at work	47
9. Marital reconciliation	45
10. Retirement	45
11. Change in health of family member	44
12. Pregnancy	40
13. Sex difficulties	39
14. Gain of new family member	39
15. Business readjustment	39
16. Change in financial state	38
17. Death of a close friend	37
18. Change to a different line of work	36
19. Change in the number of arguments with spouse	35
20. Mortgage over $60,000	31
21. Foreclosure of mortgage or loan	30
22. Change in responsibilities at work	29
23. Son or daughter leaving home	29
24. Trouble with in-laws	29
25. Outstanding personal achievement	28
26. Spouse begins or stops work	26
27. Begin or end school	26
28. Change in living conditions	25
29. Revision of personal habits	24
30. Trouble with the boss	23
31. Change in work hours or conditions	20
32. Change in residence	20
33. Change in schools	20
34. Change in recreation	19
35. Change in church activities	19
36. Change in social activities	18
37. Mortgage or loan of less than $60,000	17
38. Change in the number of family get-togethers	15
39. Change in sleeping habits	15
40. Change in eating habits	15
41. Single person living alone	10
42. Other—describe*	—

*Assign a value to events not listed above using the scores of events you feel are comparably stressful for you. *(continued)*

Test Your Stress Level *(continued)*

ANALYSIS

• **If your score totals 300 or more,** you can assume that
you've had significant amounts of stress in your life over the last
12 months. If that is the case, you would be wise to postpone
making any unnecessary decisions or changes in your life for
a while, since the stress you've been through may affect your
ability to evaluate your opinions clearly. Consider cultivating
some new stress-handling habits (see pages 45–47).

• **If your score falls below 300,** it doesn't mean that you
haven't experienced some major upheavals, but rather, that
those events have been unattended by other complications.
Stress management skills may still be important for you.

• **If your score is 100 or below,** *and* you're dissatisfied with
your life (you feel like it's stale or humdrum, or that you're
locked into a situation that for you is a dead end, personally or
professionally), it may be time for a change of some sort.
Remember: all stress is not bad! Consider a change in your
social activities, personal habits, work responsibilities, etc.
to keep yourself fresh and lively.

Are You a Type A Personality?

You've probably heard about Type A personalities and how they
are highly prone to heart disease. To assess your personality,
put checkmarks where you think your personality falls between
each pair of opposed traits. Total the numerical score indicated
by your checkmarks and find out how close you are to a true
Type A below. If you find an A-type tendency, examine your
stress management skills and fitness level to lower your
odds of trouble.

Scores
1 2 3 4 5 6 7

1. Doesn't mind leaving things temporarily unfinished ———————— Must get things finished once started

2. Calm and unhurried about appointments ———————— Never late for appointments

3. Not competitive ———————— Highly competitive

4. Listens well, lets others finish speaking ———————— Anticipates others in conversation (nods, interrupts, finishes sentences for the other)

5. Never in a hurry, even when pressured ———————— Always in a hurry

6. Able to wait calmly ———————— Uneasy when waiting

(continued)

Are You a Type A? *(continued)*

	1 2 3 4 5 6 7	
7. Slow paced	——————————	Always going full speed ahead
8. Takes one thing at a time	——————————	Tries to do more than one thing at a time, thinks about what to do next
9. Slow and deliberate in speech	——————————	Vigorous and forceful in speech (uses a lot of gestures)
10. Concerned with satisfying himself, not others	——————————	Wants recognition by others for a job well done
11. Slow doing things	——————————	Fast doing things (eating, walking, etc.)
12. Easygoing	——————————	Hard driving
13. Expresses feelings openly	——————————	Holds feelings in
14. Has a large number of interests	——————————	Few interests outside work
15. Satisfied with job	——————————	Ambitious, wants quick advancement on job
16. Never sets own deadlines	——————————	Often sets own deadlines
17. Feels limited responsibility	——————————	Always feels responsible
18. Never judges things in terms of numbers	——————————	Often judges performance in terms of numbers (how many, how much)
19. Casual about work	——————————	Takes work very seriously (works weekends, brings work home)
20. Not very precise	——————————	Very precise (careful about detail)

Total ——————

ANALYSIS

Total score 110-140: Type A_1. If you are over 40 and smoke, you are likely to have a high risk of developing cardiac illness.

Total score 80-109: Type A_2. Your risk is not as high as the A_1, but you should reduce your stress levels.

Total score 60-79: Type AB. You are a mixture of A and B patterns. This is a healthier pattern than either A_1 or A_2, but you have the potential for slipping into A behavior and you should recognize this.

Total score 30-59: Type B_2. Your behavior is on the less cardiac-prone end of the spectrum. You are generally relaxed and cope adequately with stress.

Total score 0-29: Type B_1. You tend to the extreme of non-cardiac traits. Your behavior expresses few of the reactions associated with cardiac disease.

Prepared by Dr. Howard I. Glazer, director of behavior management systems at EHE Stresscontrol Systems, Inc. Reprinted with permission of Augsburg Publishing House.

Self-Test for Stress Signals

People who manage stress well read their stress signals clearly and know when they're getting too much. Then they know what to do about it!

	Almost always	Frequently	Sometimes	Infrequently	Almost never
1. I prevent anxiety from interfering with my daily schedule	1	2	3	4	5
2. I can relax my mind and body without nicotine, alcohol or other drugs	1	2	3	4	5
3. I value my achievements	1	2	3	4	5
4. I get a sufficient amount of sleep	1	2	3	4	5
5. I am satisfied with my life	1	2	3	4	5
6. I fall asleep within 20 minutes	1	2	3	4	5
7. I have a restful night's sleep	1	2	3	4	5
8. I allow myself time to eat	1	2	3	4	5
9. I keep my mind and body in control at a comfortable pace	1	2	3	4	5
10. I make decisions easily	1	2	3	4	5

Total _____

ANALYSIS

Total score 10–19: You are taking excellent care of yourself.

Total score 20–29: You are treating your *body* well, but there are some stress signals you should become aware of.

Total score 30–39: You need to pay more attention to your stress signals.

Total score 40–50: You should re-evaluate your lifestyle and examine your stress management habits. (See pages 45–48.)

• **Eustress,** the right amount of stress, gives you a sense of mental alertness, high motivation, improved memory and recall, sharp insight, good relations with others, and a feeling that "all systems are go."

• **Distress,** an overload of stress, gives you a sense of irritability, apathy and indifference, diminished memory and recall, strained relationships, poor judgment, fatigue and insomnia.

Emotions and events

Some persons may have difficulty in taking that all-important first step to understanding the role of their emotions in their responses to events. In Kari's situation, her gut or emotional feelings are often so much more intense and persuasive than her trained rational perceptions that she blindly trusts them—even though they are causing her and others great distress. Her behavior is based on her inaccurate, emotion-laden perceptions of events at home and at the hospital.

Bill suffers from similar misperceptions. He finds it much easier to assume that the reason he drinks so much is his *work,* his *boss* or his *wife*—not himself. Bill and other abusers of alcohol perceive the trouble is "outside," not "inside," themselves.

His situation reminds me of the classic story of the alcoholic who went to his doctor.

Doctor: "Why do you drink so much, Charlie?"
Patient: "Because I'm depressed all the time."
Doctor: "Why are you depressed all the time?"
Patient: "Because I drink so much."

Positive, neutral and negative responses to events

Both Bill and Kari have spent their lives perceiving things and feeling them reflexively, in the way they *learned* as children and young adults. Their problem now is to *unlearn* that way and discover more productive ways to respond to events. They need to begin being more aware of their evaluative thoughts, that is, their tendency to interpret events with positive or, in their case, negative casts.

Most events are neutral, but people learn early in their lives to assign values to them without much intermediate thinking. People who learn to evaluate most experiences as *neutral*— or better yet, as *positive*—feel less stress. The stages, or steps, in evaluative thinking are labeled A, B and C.

• **Step A:** receiving a stimulus from the outside world: a comment from somebody, an event or something you read.

• **Step B:** forming your evaluation: positive, neutral or negative. This step is where *you* gain or lose control of your response, depending on how well you test your perceptions with outside knowledge or "self-talk." If you skip over Step B entirely and your untested evaluation is negative, you may trigger an invalid "flight-fight" response of fear or anger and subject yourself to unnecessary stress.

• **Step C:** responding to your evaluation. Negative evaluations trigger flight-fight responses: increased pulse rates, rapid breathing, sweating, a panicky feeling. Neutral evaluations require no particular response unless the situation itself requires action (you must make a reply or do something else). Positive evaluations make you feel good and may even give you a lift.

Making better evaluations

Admittedly most events are not simple and clear-cut but with this A–B–C method they are often not complex either. There are many ways of coping with situations at home or on the job that can bring you to neutral or even positive perceptions.

• **Alter your interpretation of the situation.** If you have done your best but the outcome wasn't what you expected, accept the results philosophically ("win a few, lose a few," "learn by making mistakes," "I'm not going to let it bother me"). On the other hand, don't worry about the things over which you have no control. Such worry is useless and self-destructive.

• **Change the circumstances.** This is another common method of coping. Many elements of a job, marriage or friendship can be improved by analyzing the trouble and fixing it up. The key here is clear, accurate analysis—not emotion-laden labeling.

• **Increase your threshold for distress.** Stay fit, get plenty of sleep, seek the help and support of others, pray, talk problems out.

Rational Self-Test for Threats and Problems

Cavemen, we are told, kept themselves on constant alert to danger by perceiving themselves to be constantly threatened—which they were. Modern people, however, learn to keep their nerves on constant alert not because of such *real* threats as much as from *invented* or perceived threats. This faulty pattern eventually wears them down. They need to learn which saber-toothed tigers are real and worth running from—or at least dealing with.

Such insight and priority-setting is learned with practice, and anyone can master those skills. The secret is to learn to look at troubling situations that seem to require action on your part and to give yourself this Rational Self-Test about the problem.

1. Is your perception valid and based on *objective* facts and events?   Yes____   No____

2. Will the action you plan to take protect you from probable harm?   Yes____   No____

3. Will this action help you achieve short- and long-term life goals?   Yes____   No____

4. Will this action help avoid significant emotional conflict with *others*?   Yes____   No____

5. Will this action help avoid significant emotional conflict with, and negative feelings about, *yourself*?   Yes____   No____

If, after conducting such an analysis of the event, you can answer "yes" to three of these five questions, then, *and only then,* is the situation truly threatening enough for you to evaluate your plans to take action. If you're like most modern people, you will find that the things you are busy running from only get one or two "yes" answers. Most are really only *perceived threats,* not actual threats—and there's a big difference!

• **Avoid the trouble.** This is a wise and time-honored way of coping when your other efforts fail. Recognize your limitations, and within these boundaries, set realistic goals and guidelines for yourself and others. Stay away from problematic situations or people.

Changing bad emotional habits

Use the technique of creative visualization to change bad emotional habits, that is, to avoid assigning negative evaluations to events.

• **Use your mind's eye for relief** when the pressure (or the anger) builds up. Visualize the same situation in a different way.

• **Think of other endings and other feelings.** Write your own mental script about other possible interpretations and endings for the situation.

• **Act in response to your new script,** and you'll avoid negative evaluations of events. With practice, neutral or positive evaluations will become more habitual than negative ones.

One Event — Three Responses

Let's look at an event and see it evaluated from three perspectives: negative, neutral and positive. In each case the actual event is the *same:* a hiker comes upon a nonpoisonous snake crossing the path. But the evaluation and response change, correspondingly. The point is that you can shape your response to events!

Negative perspective

- Step A: sensory perception (snake is seen).
- Step B: evaluative thought (from childhood, the hiker was told all snakes are dangerous).
- Step C: emotional response (fear, which is stressful and unwarranted).

Neutral perspective

- Step A: sensory perception (snake is seen).
- Step B: evaluative thought (hiker knows poisonous snake is unlikely; checks snake's markings; confirms nonpoisonous, no threat).
- Step C: emotional response (none; moves on and resumes hike).

Positive perspective

- Step A: sensory perception (snake is seen).
- Step B: evaluative thinking (hiker has never seen a rainbow snake in these parts).
- Step C: emotional response (interest, pleasure in observation; stays to watch and learn more).

Where to find help for handling stress

- **Family and friends.** They may tend to take your part against the outside world too much to be valuable as objective observers, but they also will be more caring listeners, and talking things out will probably help a good deal.

- **Ministers, rabbis, counselors.** These people have special skills and experience in dealing with people's problems in general, and may be able to offer new insights and perspectives for you to consider.

- **"Hot" lines.** Your white and yellow pages will have listings for crisis intervention centers with 24-hour phone answering services.

- **Medical professionals** are increasingly broad-minded about treating the whole patient. Your health care partner may also be able to refer you to other professionals who more particularly address stress-related concerns and problems.

Stress in Your Surroundings

In addition to changing your perceptions, there are many various modifications in your environment—your surroundings—that you can do to make your workplace or home less stressful.

Human engineering

There is now a special field of study, human engineering, in which architects and others coordinate architectural design and working conditions so that both mesh with the capacities and requirements of the workers. These engineers consider sound and light levels, temperature levels, air quality and the space allotted to each worker. You can evaluate your own working and living conditions as well. Ask yourself these questions.

- **Does your work or living space "feel wrong"** in any way? Analyze just how it bothers you (the charts on pages 49 and 50 will help identify typical problems). Problem indicators: inability to concentrate, constant irritations or interruptions, lack of escape space for cooling down.

- **How severe is the problem?** It could be a very minor problem, but *very* irritating, to work near a dripping faucet—and it's a problem that can be solved in 10 minutes.

- **Who can help you solve the problem?** You may need no help at all; you may need to form a committee or hold a family council to lay down new ground rules; you may have to appoint yourself as a lobbyist to promote legislation.

Mind and Body Relaxers

Whatever you choose to do as your relaxer—yoga-like exercises, meditation or transcendental meditation (TM), autogenic training, the relaxation response or a mixture of these

Stress Producing Conditions

The following lists of problems and possible solutions for them will help you identify and deal with unnecessary stress-producing conditions in your workspace. Turn to the worksheet on page 50 for help in completing your plans.

Problems	Solutions
Noise levels	
☐ Loud, continuous noises	Earplugs, sound barriers
☐ Sudden, startling noises	Schedules for quiet time
☐ Constant low drone, talk	"White noise", earplugs
☐ TV set or radio noise	Rules for family use of TV or radio
☐ Lawn mowers and other outside noise	Discuss problem with neighbors, construction crews
☐ Kids' play or teenagers' conversations	Establish play time, phone use rules
Light levels	
☐ Insufficient light	Arrange for supplementary lighting
☐ Shadowed work surface/area	Reposition light sources
☐ Overly bright light	Filtration, dimming devices
☐ Hypersensitivity to fluorescent lighting	"Dilute" fluorescence with a bit of incandescent light
Temperature levels	
☐ Constant extreme (hot, cold)	Additional heating, cooling or change in dress
☐ Fluctuation in temperatures	Examine heating/cooling plant; dress flexibly
Air quality	
☐ Stuffy atmosphere	Fans, improved ventilation, occasional "fresh air breaks"
☐ Overly dry atmosphere	Humidifier, standing water, plants
☐ Pollutants, irritants	Get protective eye, mouth and skin coverings; reduce source of irritants; increase pollution-removing efforts
Space allocation	
☐ Inadequate space	Remove all unnecessary objects to another area; increase space allotment
☐ Inefficient use of space	Study work patterns and rearrange space to meet needs

Stress Reduction Worksheet

Problems	**Solutions**
1. Noise levels	_____
	_____
	_____
	_____
	_____
2. Light levels	_____
	_____
	_____
	_____
	_____
3. Temperature levels	_____
	_____
	_____
	_____
	_____
4. Air quality	_____
	_____
	_____
	_____
	_____
5. Space allocation	_____
	_____
	_____
	_____
	_____

methods — you should know that all the well-known methods of relaxation act in a similar way. They all act on the Autonomic Nervous System (ANS) and help restore its equilibrium.

The ANS controls all the automatic systems in our body, such as appetite, sleep, body temperature, basal metabolism and so on. It also controls the primitive "flight-fight" response that is instinctual and necessary in response to threats.

The ANS helped our ancestors survive—and it helps us survive, though as we have seen, many people habitually perceive non-existent threats and overactivate that mechanism. Unless people can break these habits and let off pressure with various types of relaxation training, they end up with a variety of stress-induced illnesses such as high blood pressure, peptic ulcers and alcoholism.

There are two branches of the ANS, the sympathetic and the parasympathetic. A simplified concept of their relationship and their involvement in relaxation is shown below.

Meditation

Meditation has been called the fourth state of consciousness by some observers (following sleep, dreaming and working). It is taught in a variety of ways through transcendental meditation (TM), Zen, autogenic training, progressive relaxation and

How Relaxation Affects Your Nerves

When stress affects you, your sympathetic nervous system "overworks"—your pulse, respiration rate and blood pressure are likely to soar. In relaxation, your parasympathetic nervous system takes charge and depresses these vital signs. Consequently, following relaxation, you return to a state—and sense—of equilibrium.

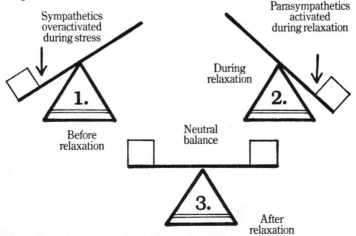

Sympathetics overactivated during stress

Parasympathetics activated during relaxation

During relaxation

1.

2.

Before relaxation

Neutral balance

3.

After relaxation

hypnosis with deep relaxation. These methods all share four basic necessities.

- **A quiet environment.**
- **A mental device** such as a sound or word (mantra).
- **A passive, accepting attitude** for relaxation.
- **A comfortable position** to keep muscular effort at a minimum.

Transcendental meditation

The mantra meditational method, popularly called TM, was originated by Maharishi Mahesh Yogi. TM is the most successful meditation system and today claims millions of adherents. Scientific studies have shown that TM produces many measurable effects such as slowed pulse, lowered blood pressure, reduced oxygen consumption and so on.

- **To learn to do TM,** you can take a six-part course offered by the International Meditation Society (there are nearly 400 teaching centers in the U.S.). Or you can read *Transcendental Meditation,* by Maharishi Mahesh Yogi (New American Library, 1973); this book outlines the basics of TM.

- **On your own,** you can simply relax for two 20-minute periods a day while you repeat a *mantra,* a syllable of your choice, and meditate. It's not really "far out" at all, and can pay off in refreshing and relaxing you.

How to Meditate

It doesn't take an extensive course in meditation skills or a period of study with your personal guru to get started—and begin getting the benefits of—meditating. If you simply follow the steps and tips below, you'll be ready to begin.

1. Find a quiet place where you can sit or lie in a position that leaves your muscles untensed. Avoid meditating for two hours after meals; the slow-down you are attempting to induce in your mind and body interferes with digestion.

2. Close your eyes and deliberately relax the muscles of your body, one by one. Most people start with their toes and work their way upward.

3. As you do this, breathe deeply through your nose.

4. When you are completely relaxed, begin saying a single word (like "one") slowly to yourself, over and over. This is your mantra. Its purpose is to focus your attention on—essentially—nothing. Try to blot out all other thoughts; continue breathing deeply.

5. After about 20 minutes of this kind of meditation (you may have to build up to it), you can stop saying the mantra and rest quietly for a few moments before opening your eyes. Then after a few more moments of relaxation, you'll be set to resume your day-to-day life.

Relaxation response

Dr. Herbert Benson, a cardiologist at Harvard, began studies in the 1970s that were designed to study the effects of transcendental meditation on hypertension. He also studied Zen, yoga, autogenic training and other relaxation methods. In the course of his work, Benson noted that a regular program of meditation along the lines of TM could be successfully used to lower blood pressure.

• **For a mantra,** he recommended using the word *one*, which he said was just as useful as the more exotic words used in TM and some other techniques. The details are outlined in his best-selling book, *Relaxation Response* (William Morrow and Co., 1975).

Yoga

Yoga is a philosophy that originated in India about 6,000 years ago. There are several forms of yoga: Gnana (spiritual), Bhakti (emotional) and Raja (mental). The one most commonly practiced in the West is Hatha (physical). Hatha Yoga was brought to Europe and America by British soldiers and civil servants one hundred years ago when they returned from service in India.

During the last 15 to 20 years, Hatha Yoga has achieved great popularity in the United States and Canada. A typical class in Hatha Yoga consists of performing deep breathing and exercises while standing, kneeling, sitting or lying on back or front. For every posture, there is a counter-posture. After about an hour, the students may be led into meditation or the teacher may give a short talk.

Try this yoga exercise as a starter.

• **Find a time of day** when there are no other distractions (phone calls, children's needs).

• **Wear comfortable, loose-fitting clothing.**

• **Set the scene.** Spread a large towel or blanket on the floor; turn down the lights; turn off the radio or TV.

• **Lie on your back,** as flat as possible, with your arms out at your sides, palms up.

• **Breathe deeply** and concentrate on relaxing your entire body for about 3 minutes.

• **Then slowly raise your hands above your head** (still touching the floor) until they meet above your head, inhaling deeply (count to eight: one-and, two-and . . .).

• **Hold your breath** (again count to eight slowly) while your hands are overhead; then exhale slowly while returning your arms to your sides (once more counting to eight). Repeat this sequence 20 times.

Positive imaging and autogenic training

Positive mental programming has always been a part of medicine and the healing arts, but the scientific basis came out of work in France that began about a century ago. Emil Coué developed the concept of auto-suggestion and worked with it, along with some standard hypnotic methods. Similar clinical applications of these techniques in the United States and Germany led to the creation of autogenic training. People do positive imaging (seeing with their mind's eye), while lying comfortably on their backs with arms at sides and legs uncrossed. They learn to relax

Relaxation Rituals

Use these suggestions to build a relaxation ritual to suit your own needs.

Homemaker	Office or Factory Worker	Child/Teen
Morning:		
Get up early to allow time for yourself before the family's needs are urgent. Read the paper, jog, bathe.	Get up early to allow enough time for paper, breakfast, family time and trip to work without rushing.	Have the next day's clothes and school gear laid out before going to bed. Eat breakfast before going to school.
Make brown-bag lunches the night before.	Write project list; start with hardest task in early morning.	
Avoid coffee, tea, cola.	Avoid coffee, tea, cola.	Avoid coffee, tea, cola.
Nap or relax along with preschoolers.	Take a break that is specifically designed for concentrated relaxation.	
Midday:		
Use lunch break as a real treat, a slow-down time. Play a favorite record; arrange your light lunch attractively; put your feet up or lie down, and visualize a favorite, peaceful place.	Avoid business lunches, booze. Several days a week, take light lunches in your office; then put your feet up or lie down, visualize a favorite spot and do some deep breathing. Finish off with a quick, cold face-wash.	After lunch at school, relax with a book or in small talk with one or two friends. On a nice day, sit out in the sun and enjoy the fresh air.
Late Afternoon/Evening:		
Before the rush of the evening meal, find quiet time and read a favorite book or watch a light-action TV program. Take a walk with the family pet.	Change clothes. Get out of work clothing, shower and change into comfortable clothes. If tense and uptight, sing loudly. Talk to the kids. Take a brisk walk to clear your head.	Get some vigorous exercise (running, biking, games, sports) after school. Talk to parents and friends about school events. After homework, take some down-time with favorite TV show, book or music.

certain muscle groups and call to mind selected visual and auditory imagery that influence moods and mental activity.

Some medical researchers have worked with the effects of imaging on such diseases as cancer and hemophilia. The validity of some of these efforts is questioned by some, but fewer and fewer physicians are prepared to roundly condemn these and other explorations of imaging as unproductive. You can experiment with the effects of imaging on your emotional state.

• **When you are anxious,** find a quiet place at work or home. Close your eyes and imagine you are at one of your favorite places or vacation spots.

• **Explore the place mentally.** Try to remember every detail: the scenery, the furniture, the sidewalks or pathways. Imagine the green of the forest until you can *see* it. Remember the *smell* of the food you cooked or ate. Recall the *sound* of the birds or the *music.* Make it all so real that you seem to be there.

• **When your mind has exhausted every detail,** you'll probably find you are calmer. Use your imagination for a quick break whenever you please.

Individualized relaxation rituals

As we discussed earlier in this section, many people develop their own mixture of relaxation methods and create their own stress-reducing rituals. By developing a routine series of symbolic actions, you can learn to step into a new role—much like an actor can do.

In stress control, the role you should assume is that of an easy-going, relaxed person, not the tense one you may be inclined to be. Athletes and musicians use similar methods to get themselves "ready." You may have heard the saying: "Even Mother Nature loves a ritual. That's why we have seasons."

• **Before developing your relaxation ritual,** identify your daily "pressure points" so you can build appropriate patterns around them. Does the morning rush of dressing, grabbing breakfast and dashing out the door set your teeth on edge? Experiment with variations until you find a more satisfying pattern.

• **Once your ritual is established,** don't get so compulsive about it that you become upset by the inevitable changes that will occur in it from time to time.

Stress resources

• Meyer Friedman and Ray H. Rosenman, *Type A Behavior and Your Heart* (Fawcett Books, 1974).

• Maxie C. Maultsby, Jr., *Help Yourself to Happiness* (Rational Self-Help Books, Lexington, Kent., 1978).

• Kenneth R. Pelletier, *Mind as Healer, Mind as Slayer* (Dell, 1977).

• Keith W. Sehnert, *Stress/ Unstress* (Augsburg, 1981).

• Hans Selye, *The Stress of Life* (McGraw Hill, 1976).

Chapter 5

Your Body, Mind and Spirit

Few people realize today that the word *psychology* originally meant the study of the human *spirit* (or soul) and not the *mind,* as it has come to be understood by most of us (the prefix "psych" comes from the Greek myth of the goddess Psyche, the human soul). Now the soul has come to mean the spiritual part of people, including their moral aspects, warmth of feeling, nobility, courage and so on.

For most of the last several hundred years, the study of the soul has been left in the hands of philosophers and theologians, both Eastern and Western. But with science's current rediscovery of the wholeness of health and life, the spiritual nature of all people is being newly examined by physicians.

In this chapter, we'll look at the significant value a spiritual life can have for you, both in terms of health and in terms of your happiness. Then we'll concentrate on how to develop or enhance your own spiritual life —whether it's in traditional religious or secular ways.

The Whole Is the Sum of the Parts

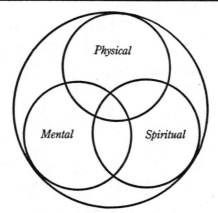

Though you cannot divide your mind from your body or your body from your spirit, it is helpful to recognize the three aspects of your nature—physical, mental, spiritual—and then consider your whole self when you examine your well-being.

Body, Mind and Spirit

A growing number of physicians and scientists are interested in the spirit, not just bodies and minds. They have come to realize that there are medical reasons, as well as religious ones, for fostering the spiritual health of their patients.

Spirituality and survival

Granger Westberg, a Lutheran hospital chaplain who worked first in Ohio and later in Illinois, has observed that some patients survived serious illnesses and stressful surgery, while others with similar medical problems did not.

- **In the survivors,** he found strengths based on spiritual values such as love, gratitude, forgiveness and hope.

- **In those who did not survive,** he found a lack of spiritual resources and, instead, negative attitudes based on anger, hate, envy and helplessness.

Church life and health

Several church-related benefits to health have been discovered in this country.

- **Regular attendance.** Among people studied in Maryland, those who went to church regularly were at "significantly less risk of dying from heart disease than those who went irregularly."

- **Social connections.** Among adults studied in Alameda County, California, the "healthiest of the healthy" were people who had good social connections

The Value of an Aesthetic or Spiritual Life

The following list names a wide variety of people who have pursued a life's work centered on aesthetic or spiritual values. In many cases, this work has fostered contentment and a general sense of well-being in the person's life—often leading to a significantly longer than average lifespan. Consider the comparable benefits that time devoted to aesthetic or spiritual concerns can bring to your own life.

- Mother Teresa
- Dr. Albert Schweitzer
- Pablo Picasso
- Helen Hayes
- Carl Sandburg
- Arthur Fiedler
- Norman Rockwell
- Rev. Jeannette Piccard
- Arthur Rubenstein
- Georgia O'Keefe
- Buckminster Fuller
- Pablo Casals

related to marriage, contacts with relatives and close friends, church or synagogue memberships, and memberships in clubs and associations.

- **Family life.** The predominantly Mormon inhabitants of Utah are much healthier than citizens of Nevada. Given the similarity of all other factors (income, schooling, degree of urbanization, climate, number of doctors and so on), the markedly better health of people in Utah, with its predominance of Mormons, seems due to their more stable family lives, abstention from tobacco and alcohol, strong family and neighborhood support, and the spiritual resources they draw from the Church of Jesus Christ of Latter-Day Saints.

• **The lesson:** people with active spiritual and social connections are healthier and happier!

Personal benefits of the spiritual life

History and literature (both secular and religious), are filled with examples of how spiritual strength has helped to sustain people through severe difficulties.

• **Viktor Frankl,** an Austrian Jew who was imprisoned in Auschwitz by the Nazis, explained how he kept up his appearance and spirits by shaving every day, even though he had to shave with bits of razors and pieces of glass. He kept up hope by imagining how he would spend his time with his wife, family and friends when he got out of the concentration camp.

• **Kathryn Koob,** one of the two American women who were held as hostages by Iran and then dramatically released on President Reagan's inaugural day, told of using prayers to strengthen her spirit throughout the long ordeal.

• **General Jonathan Wainwright** survived the Bataan deathmarch and three years of imprisonment by the Japanese in the Philippines from 1942–45 by reciting bits of prayers and encouraging other captives to do the same. He survived and took part in the surrender of the Japanese delegates aboard the U.S.S. *Missouri* in Tokyo Bay.

• **The lesson:** a strong spiritual life can help you through adversities.

Right Brain, Left Brain and Spirituality

Additional insights about human behavior and human nature — and perhaps the spirit — have come from studies during the last decade about the differences between the right and left halves of the brain. According to these studies, the two halves have the following characteristics.

Left Half
• analytical
• used for narrow-focus activities
• verbal thinking
• right-handed coordination

Right Half
• creativity; artistic effort
• experimentation; open-ended
• non-verbal thinking; spatial thinking
• left-handed coordination
• processing dreams, films

Clearly the right half of the brain may be the side allied with the spiritual life as we tend to think of it. And it stands to reason that a fully integrated person will make full use of both sides of the brain. Do you really use yours to its full capability?

The value of forgiveness

Nobody's perfect—we all grant that. And yet when others wrong or hurt us, whether through ignorance, thoughtlessness or even malice, it often becomes difficult to forgive them and put the wrong behind us. Yet if we don't, we waste emotional and spiritual energy and generate undue stress for *ourselves,* somehow expecting repayment of a debt that cannot really be repaid. What can we do?

• **Make sure** that the hurt is not of your own making. That is, examine the possibility that you misunderstood or misinterpreted events—not to excuse others, but to clarify the situation rationally.

• **Evaluate** the "wrong." Was it intentional or unintentional? The more objective you can be, the fewer *intended* wrongs you will have to deal with. Unintended wrongs are easier to forgive.

• **Recognize,** as Luther did, that the faults of others are in us, "maybe not exactly the same ones, but probably worse ones."

• **Accept** the fact that if you are wronged, you may need to point out the harm to the person who's harmed you. Doing so may still not repair the damage, but may help you to let go of your hurt. As Blake wrote, "I was angry with my friend,/I told my wrath and my wrath did end."

• **Consider** the possibility that you might have done similar wrong in a similar situation.

Try to put yourself in the other person's shoes. Rising above another's failure may ease the transition from hurt to forgiveness.

Spiritual experiences: who has them?

Having a spiritually active life does not necessarily mean you've had a revelation. Eugene Thomas and Pamela Cooper of the University of Connecticut studied 305 persons from all backgrounds and walks of life. They asked this question: "Have you ever had the feeling of being close to a powerful spiritual force that seemed to lift you outside of yourself?"

• **One person in three (34%)** noted an intense spiritual experience. This percentage is similar to other studies in the United States (35%) and Britain (36%).

• **But only 3 people out of 100 (3%)** reported intense spiritual experiences that produced awesome emotions and a feeling of oneness with God, nature or the universe. Afterward, these people changed their perceptions of time and surroundings, had a feeling of "knowing" more and as a result, reordered the priorities of their life. They became more flexible in their attitudes than those who had not had such an experience.

• **Most people,** therefore, live on a lower spiritual plane than those who have intense spiritual experiences. But we can "make do" and cultivate a spiritual or aesthetic sense, enjoying its benefits nevertheless.

Spirituality and death

This same type of flexible attitude toward life and reordering of priorities has been reported by people who have had near-death experiences. Investigators such as Elizabeth Kübler-Ross, Raymond Moody and Kenneth Ring have found that when they talked to persons who had had a brush with death following an accident, critical illness or suicide attempt, the survivors reported several typical changes.

• **Increased acceptance of others** and more and more compassion for them.

• **Increased willingness to love** others more openly.

• **Diminished fear** of death.

Ring concluded, "Perhaps one lesson to realize is that there is indeed a higher spiritual dimension that pervades our lives and that we will discover it for ourselves in the moment of death. The question is, however, will we discover it in the moments of our lives?"

Spiritual activities

Throughout life, most of us are exposed to activities that can enrich our spiritual lives. This enrichment can come from a wide variety of experiences, religious and secular.

• **Hearing religious or classical music** performed by orchestras, choirs, soloists or organists.

• **Seeing works of art** with a religious or spiritual significance such as tapestries, wood carvings, sculptures and paintings.

How's Your Spiritual Life?

When was the last time you (check one that applies):

	Yesterday or today	Last week	Last month	Last year	Don't remember
1. Shared 10 minutes with a child and talked about a common interest?					
2. Went to regular church, synagogue or religious service?					
3. Helped someone who is less fortunate (in your opinion) than you?					
4. Took a walk in the park or woods with someone you love?					

(continued)

How's Your Spiritual Life? *(continued)*

	Yesterday or today	Last week	Last month	Last year	Don't remember
5. Prayed for someone?					
6. Watched the sun come up (or go down) while at a lake, in the mountains, in the woods, at home or wherever you might be?					
7. Went to a special church, synagogue or religious service (or served on church committees, programs or related service)?					
8. Read the Bible or related inspirational or devotional materials?					
9. Spent 15–30 minutes meditating, praying, pondering or reflecting on your purpose in life?					
10. Attended an art exhibition, a theater or dance performance or a concert featuring religious works? Or listened to religious works on a radio or stereo?					
(Score per check)	6	4	2	1	0
SUB TOTAL					
TOTAL SCORE					

ANALYSIS

After totaling your score, take a look at the general guidelines for interpreting results below.

Score	Interpretation
40–60	You should be enjoying all the benefits of a spiritually rich life.
30–39	You have a good emphasis on spiritual values in your life.
20–29	Spiritual concerns are a part of your life, but you may want to spend more time concentrating on them.
0–19	Your spiritual life is underdeveloped. Try to bring these values into the limelight, even if it takes some extra effort on your part.

- **Reading the Bible,** books of philosophy or devotional materials.

- **Participating in services** at one's church or synagogue.

- **Praying** or meditating.

- **Experiencing the beauty** of a lake, mountain, meadow or forest.

- **Helping a friend** or family member in times of trouble.

Spiritual rituals

When an activity stirs your soul or refreshes your spirit, be sure to repeat the event on a *regular* basis. Establish traditions or rituals that enhance the experience.

- **Attend not only the special services** at your church or synagogue, but also the regular services.

- **Go to worship 15 minutes early** to hear the organ prelude. Enjoy it!

- **Learn more about art.** When you hear that your local museum has a new art show or exhibition, take extra time to study the literature about it so you can appreciate it fully. Go on the guided tour to further deepen your understanding.

- **Complement your reading of the Bible with commen-** tary and supplements by capable scholars who can provide insight and background.

- **Set aside a regular time each day** for prayer or meditation. Do it when you are unhurried and fresh. Don't wait until you are so tired that you can barely keep your mind—and eyes—open.

- **Try to take time off** to "commune with nature" at least once a week. You will find it will refresh your soul to walk in a park, stroll by a lake or sit in the forest. If you're a city-dweller, create a corner of your apartment for meditation with plants, soothing furnishings and so on.

- **Establish a goal** that it is better use of your time to collect people than to collect material things: help a friend, counsel a family member, listen to a fellow worker. It will pay off in many ways.

Spiritual resources

- Bradley Hanson, *The Call of Silence* (Augsburg, 1980).

- W. Brugh Joy, *Joy's Way* (J. B. Tarcher, 1979).

- George Ritchie with Elizabeth Sherrill, *Return from Tomorrow* (Chosen Books, 1978).

Chapter 6

Controlling Hazards in Your Surroundings

A recent trip to the Los Angeles area gave me first-hand experience about the impact one's surroundings can have on one's health. The sounds, smells, sights and space limitations my mind and body were subjected to gave me ample proof that adverse surroundings take their toll on people.

My body needed no additional convincing about the bad effects of high-decibel traffic noise, air pollution, unpleasant sights and cramped personal space. How did I react to the roar of traffic on Interstate 5 from Anaheim to downtown Los Angeles, to the deafening air hammers used in construction at the UCLA campus, even to the irritation of the loud rock music coming from a teenager's portable radio at Disneyland?

As modern-day city dwellers often do, I grew nervous, tense and irritable—and in three days, I got sick! These conditions are *bad* for you. So in this chapter, you'll find ways you can minimize the impact of these negative conditions on you, both at home and away.

Your Risk Profile

When you look at your age group's risk of dying from various causes, you'll notice an intriguing pattern (see below).

The Three Major Causes of Death

The table below is based on actuarial tables of the most likely causes of death for people of various ages. For each death, however, there are countless injuries and near-deaths.

Age group	White male	White female	Black male	Black female
5-9 years	Car accidents	Car accidents	Car accidents	Car accidents
	Drowning	Leukemia	Drowning	Fire accidents
	Leukemia	Fire accidents	Fire accidents	Homicide*
10-14 years	Car accidents	Car accidents	Homicide*	Homicide*
	Suicide	Homicide*	Car accidents	Car accidents
	Drowning	Suicide	Drowning	Drowning
15-19 years	Car accidents	Car accidents	Homicide*	Homicide*
	Suicide	Suicide	Car accidents	Car accidents
	Homicide*	Homicide*	Drowning	Suicide

*A high percentage of homicide deaths for those under 20 is related to child abuse.   *(continued)*

Major Causes of Death *(continued)*

Age group	White male	White female	Black male	Black female
20-24 years	Car accidents Suicide Homicide	Car accidents Suicide Homicide	Homicide Car accidents Suicide	Homicide Car accidents Suicide
25-29 years	Car accidents Suicide Homicide	Car accidents Suicide Homicide	Homicide Car accidents Suicide	Homicide Car accidents Cirrhosis
30-34 years	Car accidents Suicide Heart disease	Car accidents Suicide Breast cancer	Homicide Car accidents Heart disease	Homicide Cirrhosis Breast cancer
35-39 years	Heart disease Car accidents Suicide	Breast cancer Suicide Heart disease	Homicide Heart disease Cirrhosis	Heart disease Cirrhosis Breast cancer
40-44 years	Heart disease Lung cancer Car accidents	Breast cancer Heart disease Lung cancer	Heart disease Homicide Cirrhosis	Heart disease Breast cancer Stroke
45-49 years	Heart disease Lung cancer Cirrhosis	Heart disease Breast cancer Lung cancer	Heart disease Lung cancer Stroke	Heart disease Stroke Breast cancer
50-54 years	Heart disease Lung cancer Cirrhosis	Heart disease Breast cancer Lung cancer	Heart disease Lung cancer Stroke	Heart disease Stroke Breast cancer
55-59 years	Heart disease Lung cancer Stroke	Heart disease Breast cancer Lung cancer	Heart disease Lung cancer Stroke	Heart disease Stroke Breast cancer
60-64 years	Heart disease Lung cancer Stroke	Heart disease Stroke Breast cancer	Heart disease Lung cancer Stroke	Heart disease Stroke Diabetes
65-69 years	Heart disease Lung cancer Stroke	Heart disease Stroke Breast cancer	Heart disease Stroke Lung cancer	Heart disease Stroke Diabetes
70-74 years	Heart disease Stroke Lung cancer	Heart disease Stroke Intestinal & Rectal cancer	Heart disease Stroke Lung cancer	Heart disease Stroke Diabetes

Note: This table is based on data from the Department of Prospective Medicine, Methodist Hospital of Indiana, Indianapolis, Indiana.

Up to the age of about 30, the leading causes of death tend to be people-related: automobile accidents, suicides, homicides (including deaths from child abuse) and drownings are largely responsible for the deaths of younger people. After 30, those causes of fatalities decline and illnesses begin to have their impact.

It's not a pleasant subject, but to put it positively, you stand a *real* chance of improving your odds of survival past 30 if you pay particular attention to those risks you can control: your car driving habits, including use of seat belts for yourself and your children; your care in storing weapons so they're neither stolen nor seized in a moment of anger. And if you've survived your thirtieth birthday, then your already healthy lifestyle (with attention to fostering your fitness of body, mind and spirit) can improve your odds of a long, healthy life.

Your Home Environment

More accidents occur at home than anywhere else. Most of us spend about 12 hours a day there, so it's well worth a look at the home front when you realize its direct impact on your health.

Pollutants, toxins, hazards

Consider some of the chemicals you frequently use around the house—benzene, naphtha, chlo-rinated hydrocarbons, aromatic nitrates and so on. Also consider the materials that surround you —formaldehyde (in insulation), asbestos, carbon monoxide. What can you do about these substances, without even knowing for sure that they are hazardous to you?

• **Make it your business to be informed.** Keep abreast of the growing fund of knowledge about household hazards. This may mean some effort, for instance, writing to the manufacturer of your hair dryer to find out if the model you've been using for years was made with asbestos.

• **Read labels on products thoroughly** to learn what techniques you must use—for safety's sake.

• **Don't use certain products or foods** that have been proven to contain harmful ingredients.

• **Make your own home cleaners** to avoid the costly supercleaners on the supermarket shelves. They will be safer to use. (See page 68.)

Home safety information

For more information about home safety, write to the sources below.

• Aetna Life and Casualty Insurance Company, 151 Farmington Ave., Hartford, CT 06115.

• National PTA, 700 North Rush St., Chicago, IL 60611.

• National Safety Council, 425 North Michigan Ave., Chicago, IL 60611.

• Safety Now, P.O. Box 567, Jenkintown, PA 19046.

• U.S. Consumer Product Safety Commission, Washington, DC 20207.

Accidental Poisoning Prevention

There are several resources available to you on the subject of accidental poisoning of children. One information resource is the National Poison Center Network, 125 DeSoto Street, Pittsburgh, PA 15213 (412-681-6669). By contacting them, you can learn the telephone number of the U.S. poison control center nearest you. For poison control information in Canada, contact the Department of Health and Welfare, Brooke Clarton Blvd., Ottawa, Ontario K1A 0K9 (613-992-0979). Add this number to your Emergency Telephone Numbers Form (see page 93) and keep it by your phone. You can also have the Network send you a dozen Mr. Yuk stickers and a home teaching unit on poison prevention. The cost is $1, to cover postage. Place these stickers prominently on drugs, medicines and poisonous household products in your home; children react strongly to Mr. Yuk's expression!

Homemakers' risks

A 15-year study of homemakers in Oregon showed that they face a "significant excess of cancer deaths" for cancers of the breast, ovary, colon, lung, uterus and stomach. Women whose occupations lay outside the home had a 54% lower rate of death from these cancers. The probable sources of the homemakers' cancer risks are these:

• toxic chemical fumes

• low-level radiation from television sets and microwave ovens

• oversmoking

• overeating

• overindulgence with alcohol

• lack of exercise

Since homemakers represent the largest single workforce in the country, it's clear that the risks they encounter touch on a significant number of people. Obviously changes in lifestyle for these people could have marked effects on their longevity. If you are a homemaker, give some thought to how you can avoid some of these hazards and restructure your working life to avoid them.

Fireproofing the home

• **Install enough smoke detectors** to adequately monitor your entire home.

• **Keep multipurpose fire extinguishers** near potential fire areas: kitchen, basement, fireplace.

• **Screen the fireplace.** Make sure a protective screen encloses the entire opening and set up fireplace-use rules for your children.

• **Conduct fire drills** regularly and plan preferred and alternate exit routes for all family members.

Hazardous Household Substances

You can find substances made from dangerous chemicals in practically every room in your house. Keep the home environment a safe place to live in by following the tips on page 65. Read the chart below for a list of specific hazardous substances with suggestions for what to do to prevent accidents from happening in your home.

Substance	Hazard	What to Do
Flammables* (solvents, such as benzene, naptha, paint thinner)	Fire caused by contact with open flame	Keep away from pilot light or flame; if close to source of flame, put out pilot light completely
Aerosols (such as hairspray, bug killers, chlorinated hydrocarbons)	Fire caused by proximity to open flame; explosion caused by heat	Never use near an open flame; never store in hot places
Food extracts (such as vanilla or maple extract)	Poisoning (if taken in undiluted form—straight from the bottle)	Keep out of reach of children
Asbestos (as in ceiling insulation)	Cancer (of the lung, lining of chest and abdomen, stomach, intestine)	Avoid buildings with known asbestos problem; cover or remove asbestos from building, if necessary
Formaldehyde (as in wall insulation)	Respiratory problems caused by inhalation of vapors	Never install insulation of this type unless it's been treated according to current safety regulations
Carbon monoxide	Poisoning by inhalation (from car exhaust, heating system, water or space heater)	Be sure that garage is sealed off from the house; keep fireplace damper open until fire is completely out; have heating system inspected once a year

*Remember to never mix these (or any other) cleaners together! Instead of making a more powerful cleaning solution, you'll be risking a serious accident or injury.

Checklist for
Safe, Cheap Cleaners

Here are some inexpensive and less hazardous household cleaning combinations that can become alternatives to the costly commercial cleaners you may now use.

☐ **Multipurpose cleaner:** Mix together ½ cup ammonia, ⅓ cup Arm and Hammer washing soda (sodium carbonate) and 1 gallon warm water.

☐ **Deodorizer:** Plain baking soda.

☐ **Drain cleaner:** ½ cup washing soda (sodium carbonate) followed by 2 cups of boiling water.

☐ **Upholstery and rug shampoo:** Mix together ¼ cup liquid dishwashing detergent, 1 cup warm water and 2 tablespoons vinegar. Beat with egg beater or mixer until stiff foam develops. Apply by scrubbing. Let dry and vacuum.

☐ **Copper cleaner:** Dip half a lemon in table salt and scrub. Rinse and buff dry for a safe shine.

☐ **Sink cleaner:** Table salt. It disinfects too.

Wood stove safety

A minor epidemic of burns caused directly and indirectly by wood-burning stoves is one unfortunate side-effect of their growing popularity. Here are a few common-sense ideas you should know if you're considering buying or have already installed a wood stove in your home.

• **Be sure the installation is safe.** Any reputable stove dealer can give you the specifications for minimum distances to flammable surfaces, and can suggest ways to fireproof the floor, walls and ceiling nearest the stove. Install a stove thermometer so you don't overheat the stove or chimney and waste fuel.

• **Make sure your chimney is safe.** This applies to its construction as well as its maintenance. You'll need a professional chimney sweeping once a year, but you can help purge some of the deposits on the walls of the chimney if you periodically throw a handful of table salt into the flames.

• **Educate your family in firecraft.** Show them how to build and tend fires that aren't overly hot, and teach children not to play with the matches.

• **Store tools and supplies safely.** Don't let children play with pokers, tongs or bellows; keep axes and hatchets out of reach.

• **Build barriers around the stove if you have toddlers.** Don't trust verbal warnings to keep their hands away from the heat; remember that you can't watch them constantly either.

Home Safety Checklist

The following checklist points out specific steps you can take to make every room in your home as safe as possible. Turn to page 70 for additional suggestions for childproofing your home.

1. Living room
☐ Screen the fireplace.
☐ Move any trailing cords.
☐ Add carpet pad so that carpet won't slip.

2. Kitchen
☐ Add pan guards to stove.
☐ Use garbage can with childproof top.
☐ Install nonslip floor surface.
☐ Hang fire extinguisher close to stove.
☐ Add locks to cupboards with hazardous substances (see page 67).

3. Stairway
☐ Install light switches at top and bottom of stairway.
☐ Remove any obstacles from stairs.
☐ Check to see that carpet runner on stairs is securely in place.

4. Bathroom
☐ Install grab bars in the tub.
☐ Lock up medicine cabinet.
☐ Make sure that mats are of the nonslip type.
☐ Locate electric outlets as far away from the tub as possible.

5. Bedroom
☐ Check to see that electric blanket is in safe condition and grounded.
☐ Keep any space heater away from curtains or furniture.

6. Child's bedroom
☐ Check to see that bed has high sides.
☐ Remove any broken or damaged toys from the room.
☐ Add safety bars to any windows.

Checklist for Childproofing

☐ Have you tucked cords safely behind kitchen appliances?

☐ Are your cleaning supplies locked up and/or out of reach from children?

☐ Is your bathroom medicine chest locked up?

☐ Do you have your children use paper or plastic drinking cups instead of breakable glass ones?

☐ Have all broken toys been thrown out?

☐ Have you covered all electrical outlets?

☐ Are plugged-in cords with excess length wound up?

☐ Have you placed eye-level decals on sliding glass doors?

☐ Do you use safety locks on drawers and cupboards?

☐ Are all childproof caps secured after use?

☐ Do you use Mr. Yuk stickers? (See page 66.)

Preventing falls

• **Keep a night light** on in bathrooms, and install grab bars in tubs.

• **Winterize outdoor steps** and porches with non-slip surfaces. When snow or ice is present, use rock salt or sand.

• **Clean up spills** dropped on floors immediately to prevent people from slipping.

• **Think twice** about buying shoes with leather soles and heels. Rubber and neoprene materials have better "grab power."

• **Carry no loads** that block your vision; require other family members to follow the same rule.

• **Keep a supply of emergency candles** and flashlights to use in case of power failures, so you won't be left groping—and tripping—in the dark.

Car Safety

We can take some small consolation from the fact that during the periods of gas shortages in the 70s, deaths on highways declined as people stayed home to conserve fuel. Unfortunately, since then the trend has reversed itself, and in 1981, over 52,000 people became fatality statistics —many of them under 30 and meeting early deaths.

Car and traffic safety are complex issues, but progress *is* being made in the product research into safer designs of cars and roadways. Nevertheless, your greatest investment in safety with automobiles comes from developing sensible driving habits.

Driving tips

• **When you shop for a car,** consider its safety rating along with its gas mileage and comfort.

• **Wear your seatbelt** and shoulder restraint *every time* you are in a moving car. Insist that all passengers do likewise.

• **Drive defensively:** anticipate the errors and lapses of other drivers, be on the lookout for road hazards, and so on. Know where every car around you is heading.

- **Obey all laws** and signs; match your driving speed to existing conditions.

- **Don't drive** when you're tired or have been drinking.

- **Take the ignition key** with you when you leave the car.

- **Keep road flares,** a first-aid kit, a fire extinguisher and a winter survival kit (if appropriate) in your car.

Cars and children

- **From birth on,** children should ride in proper restraints: a car seat, harness or belt. The March, 1975 and June, 1977 issues of *Consumer Reports* evaluate restraints. Old-fashioned "car seats" are no good.

Recommended Child Car Seats

Two child car seats that have been recommended as proper restraints are:

- Peterson Safety Shell
- GM Love Seat

Both can be obtained from Safety Now Co., Inc., P.O. Box 567, Jenkintown, PA 19046.

- **Do not allow children to play** in cars, especially with the car controls; never leave children under 12 alone in cars.

- **Don't place small children** in the seats that are closest to open windows.

- **Avoid letting children close** car doors or trunks.

- **Keep any sharp or heavy objects** in the car trunk, *not* in the back seat.

- **Don't leave an unattended car** with its motor running when children are playing nearby.

Travel Safety

Although fewer people are killed in airplane accidents than in car accidents each year, as an informed traveler you can take specific steps to protect against possible hazards or injuries. And you can apply the same smart consumerism to safety at your hotel accommodations.

Flying tips

- **Learn all that you can** about the different models of airplanes and their potential risks. Ask the airline to tell you the model of plane that you're scheduled to fly on so you know whether you're booked on a high- or low-risk flight.

- **Ask for a seat** in the nonsmoking section. There's no need to breathe in someone else's irritating smoke as you fly across the country!

- **Pay attention** while the flight attendant demonstrates the safety procedures. Be sure to locate the exit that's nearest to you.

Flying with children

- **If you have a small baby,** reserve a bassinet when you arrange for your flight. Also ask for the flight that is the least crowded—you'll be more likely to find an empty seat to put your baby in (babies under two are not assigned seats).

- **Give your baby a bottle** or pacifier at landing and takeoff time to reduce pressure on the ears. Give older children gum or hard candy.
- **Never drink hot beverages** while you hold your child in your lap. If the drink spills, the child might be scalded.

Hotel fire precautions

Recent hotel fires have highlighted the need for informed caution on the part of travelers, whether they are away from home on business or vacation trips. Follow the tips below whenever you check into a hotel; they could help you avert a tragedy.

- **Pick a safe floor.** Remember that hook-and-ladder trucks can only reach, at best, to the twelfth or thirteenth floor. If you're assigned a room that's higher than that, your escape during a blaze will probably be up through the roof or down, on foot, through the stairway. If you are not capable of climbing or descending many stairs, ask for a room on a lower floor.
- **Know the alarm system.** Ask what the hotel's fire alarm sounds like when you check in. There may also be a brochure detailing fire escape plans, so ask for one at the same time.
- **Find your exit.** When you get to your room, count the number of hallway doors to the nearest fire exit and memorize its location. In a fire, it's likely that the hall will be dark or even smoke-filled, and you may need to count doors to reach the nearest exit.

- **Try the exit door.** It may be locked from the outside, so don't get yourself locked in the stairwell! But if it's locked on the hallway side (so you can't escape), report it to the hotel management. If you're told that it's hotel policy to keep the exits locked, ask how they are unlocked in the event of a fire. If you don't get satisfactory answers, check out of the hotel—and notify the local fire department.
- **Keep your room key in the same spot** whenever you're in your room, in case you need to grab it and run. (You may be forced to return to your room during a fire if you find your escape route is blocked.)

What to do in a hotel fire

- **If you hear the fire alarm** or smell (or see) smoke, call the local fire department and *then* the front desk.
- **Stay low during a fire.** Noxious gases and smoke will concentrate above you and gradually move downward. Be prepared to *crawl.*
- **Pocket your room key and feel the door** before opening it. If it's cool, open it a crack. If the hall is not on fire, walk (or crawl) to the exit and go downstairs. If the way down is blocked, go up to the roof, a probable rescue site. If you can't get to (or through) the exit, return to your room.
- **Never use an elevator to escape a fire.** They are proven death traps.

• **If your door is hot, keep it closed,** because the hall's on fire. Don't panic, however. The tips below will help you buy time and give rescuers a chance to reach you.

When fire traps you in your room

• **Call the fire department** and tell them your location.

• **Open your window if it's not smoky outside.** Do *not* open it if you see smoke. If your window doesn't open, use a chair to break it if it's clear outside.

• **Keep smoke out of your room** by soaking towels or phone-book pages in water and using them to stuff cracks in the door, seal air vents shut and so on. If possible, use the bathroom fan to vent out the smoke.

• **Keep the room cool.** Flood the floors; throw water on the door and walls (use your ice bucket); wet the curtains.

• **Keep yourself cool.** Filter smoke with a wet towel around your face. Wrap up in a wet blanket. Stay *down,* where the cooler, clearer air is.

• **Keep up your efforts.** Help will be coming!

The Big Picture: Your Environment

It's all very well to "clean up your act" personally, adopting a healthy lifestyle and paying attention to the hazards in your home—and in that extension of your home, your car. But what about the air you breathe, the water you drink? What about your workplace, if you work outside your home?

You owe it to your health, and to the health of others, to take on a broader sense of your surroundings, because air, water and even space are our shared possessions and responsibilities. Here are a few thoughts about steps you can take to ensure the quality of your surroundings.

Get smart

• **Learn about your job's hazards**—the risks you face by virtue of working where you do. What are the most important occupational hazards and on-the-job accident risks you face daily? Electronic screens, chemical solvents (even those in office duplicating machines), gases, dust and other materials make virtually every job carry some inherent risks. And the more physically active your work is, the greater the additional risk of personal injury through accidents is to you. Be aware of the particular hazards that are a part of your day; learn to protect yourself.

• **Learn about your neighborhood's hazards.** Nobody really wants to know about these problems, but ignorance won't protect you from their effects. Are you downwind from an airborne polluter? Are toxic wastes buried miles away liable to enter the groundwater and affect your supply? Are industries moving in on precious green spaces nearby?

Get active

- **Form a COSH group** (a Committee on Occupational Health and Safety) at work to investigate and solve environmental problems in your workplace.

- **Join or form a concerned citizens' group** to tackle problems of air, water and noise pollution and safety that affect you and others.

- **Write letters** to your local newspaper editors and to elected local, regional, state and national representatives. Make your concerns their concerns, and you'll get results.

Home safety resources

- Joy M. Arena and Miriam Bachar, *Child Safety is No Accident* (Hawthorne, 1978).

- Paul Brodeur, *The Zapping of America* (W. W. Norton, 1977).

- Murl Harmon, *A New Vaccine for Child Safety* (Safety Now Co., Inc., Jenkintown, Penn., 1976).

- Jeanne M. Stellman and Susan Daum, *Work is Dangerous to Your Health* (Vintage, 1972).

Chapter 7

Getting the Best Health Care

When you think about your health-care arrangements, no doubt you picture your doctor or nurse-practitioner—your "principal health-care manager," in the language of the trade. But that person is only a small part of this country's vast health-care system. To get the most from that system, you need to be sure that your health-care manager is the best available, and you need to know how to work effectively with him or her and the system.

This chapter will set you up to find a person in the health-care system—a physician, nurse-practitioner or other health worker—who best meets your particular needs. It will also show you how to keep the actual cost of your health care down. Remember that ultimately, patients and professionals are all after the same thing: quality care at the least expense.

Choosing a Health-Care Professional

It almost goes without saying that you need a personal health manager, someone you can call your "family doctor" or "family health advisor." Whoever you use should be understanding, compassionate, skilled, sympathetic and available when you need him or her. Moreover, the style of care and implied role toward you (partner? friend? professional consultant? boss?) should be one you desire and value.

If the health-care professional you use doesn't fit that mold or if you've moved and don't have a doctor or allied health professional to work with, here are some tips on how to locate a good one. The process involves getting personal references, checking out directories and evaluating a number of candidates before you even schedule a get-acquainted interview. Take a little time for this search: it's important to find a good personal health advisor, a compatible partner for your health care.

Personal references
• **Run your own "Gallup Poll."** Phone or visit a half-dozen neighbors or relatives in the area and get their recommendations. Co-workers can help too. By the time your checking is done, you should have a good list of candidates who are worth further research.

• **Ask nurses and doctors.** The strongest recommendation for medical competence is one you get from a hospital staff nurse, intern or resident who has seen the doctor in action and can judge the doctor's abilities. Draw on social contacts with these people if you can; donate some time to a hospital to develop contacts if you haven't any. If you don't know a medical person, ask around for someone who does.

Directories

• **Use the yellow pages.** Your yellow pages may categorize doctors by their specialties, under headings like *Psychiatry* or *Surgery.* If it doesn't (it depends on how conservative your local medical society is), get the number of the county medical society.

• **Call the medical society.** The usual policy for such requests is to give out three names, chosen in an objective rotation from the membership roster. Some physicians may not even be taking on new patients, but call and find out. The local medical society will direct you to the kind of specialist or physician you want.

• **Check on a "doctors' directory."** Ask your local library or consumer protection agency if such a directory has been compiled for your community. It will provide detailed information about local physicians: office locations, credentials and affiliations, usual office and lab charges, types of billing practices, willingness to accept Medicare and Medicaid payments, types and sizes of staff and accessibility.

Checklists

When you have several candidates lined up, set up a checklist (similar to the one on pages 77–79) for each one. A phone call to each candidate should give you the answers to many of the questions the checklist covers; the rest can be taken up when you meet your "finalist(s)" in person.

• **Don't be dismayed** if the office nurse can't answer everything for you. Note, however, professionals whose treatment of prospective patients is curt or unfriendly.

• **Be cooperative** with the office nurse. If she's busy when you call, ask if you can call back or if she can return your call when things are quieter.

• **Survey your checklists** when your calls are complete and plan to visit the best candidate. In all likelihood, you'll have a single best prospect. If you have more than one, see the front-runner first. You may be so pleased with your initial contact that you won't need to see anybody else!

Meeting the candidate

• **Set up an appointment.** Now that you've got a first choice, plan a 10- to 15-minute interview for which, most likely, you'll have to pay the usual visit fee. It's still a good investment.

• **Make it clear that you're a prospective patient** and you'd like to get acquainted (oftentimes new patients are given an introductory presentation by a nurse or office aide first).

• **Bring your checklist along** and fill in the answers to any unanswered questions you have.

Checklist for Choosing a Doctor or Health-Care Professional

The following checklist should help you in identifying and narrowing down your choices of candidates for the best health-care professional you can find. If you fill in the information for your top choices, you'll be ready to compare them and decide which ones are worth a get-acquainted visit. Note: starred items are discussed in detail on pages 79–85.

1. Basic Information

Name _____

Address _____

Phone (office) _____

      (24-hour answering service) _____

Hospital affiliation(s)* _____

_____

Accepting new patients?   Yes ☐   No ☐

Type of professional* (check one)

family doctor ☐ obstetrician/gynecologist ☐
nurse-practitioner ☐ pediatrician ☐
internist (specialist in internal medicine) ☐
physician's assistant or "P.A." ☐
other specialist (type) _____

Type of practice* (check one)

solo practice ☐ group practice ☐
single-specialty group ☐ multiple-specialty group ☐

Professional affiliations* (check one or more)

teaching appointment at a university ☐
on hospital medical staff ☐
specialist (three-year internship) ☐
member of professional medical group(s) ☐

Use of paramedical professionals* (check one or more)

nurse-practitioners ☐ physicians' assistants ☐
nurse midwives ☐

2. Basic Services

	Yes	No	Don't Know
sees patients by appointment only	___	___	___
allows walk-in visits	___	___	___
practice covered at all times	___	___	___
allows at least 15 minutes per routine visit	___	___	___

(continued)

Checklist for Choosing a Doctor or Health-Care Professional *(continued)*

	Yes	No	Don't Know
thorough baseline history plus current medical records kept*	—	—	—
medical records open to patients concerned*	—	—	—
gives advice on the phone	—	—	—
1- to 5-day wait for routine visits	—	—	—
accepts senior citizens (Medicare recipients) as patients	—	—	—

3. Accessibility

bus or nearby public transportation	—	—	—
stairs to office/ramp available	—	—	—
wheelchair available	—	—	—
free parking nearby	—	—	—

4. Special Services

babysitting	—	—	—
patient-education classes offered or encouraged	—	—	—
patient-advocate services*	—	—	—
interpreter (for languages other than English, or for hearing impaired)	—	—	—

5. Medical/Laboratory Services

x-ray in building or nearby	—	—	—
minor surgery in office	—	—	—
family planning	—	—	—
treats fractures	—	—	—
blood tests	—	—	—
cardiograms	—	—	—
obstetrical care	—	—	—
casting and minor orthopedic services	—	—	—
urine tests, strep tests without full office call required*	—	—	—
proctoscopy	—	—	—
generic medications optional on prescriptions*	—	—	—

(continued)

Checklist for Choosing a Doctor or Health-Care Professional *(continued)*

6. Billing Information

	Yes	No	Don't Know
immediate payment required	—	—	—
new patient pre-payment required	—	—	—
accepts Medicare/Medicaid	—	—	—
will discuss fees and charges	—	—	—
will help prepare insurance forms	—	—	—
discount for cash payments	—	—	—

7. Medical Philosophy

The professional's positions on:

vitamins and nutrition _____

medical self-care _____

tranquilizers _____

antibiotics _____

diet pills _____

breast feeding _____

second opinions _____

other matters that concern you _____

• **Watch for style as well as content** as you and your potential health-care partner talk. Do you like this person's manner? Do you like this person's medical philosophy?

Hospital affiliations

Where does your health-care professional send patients if they need hospitalization? The kind of hospital your doctor or allied professional is affiliated with tells you something.

• If it's a **university teaching hospital,** you can assume requirements for "attending" (having staff privileges and being able to admit patients) are stiff. These professional plums must be earned, often through teaching young doctors and nurses. However, don't take this kind of affiliation as a money-back guarantee of quality, and remember that the time devoted to lectures, conferences and such may make it harder to get answers to your health-care questions.

• If your candidate is on the **staff at three or four hospitals,** think twice. The numbers may be impressive, but making rounds to them all can be detrimental to prompt patient care. The doctor could be in surgery at Hospital C when you're in post-surgical shock at Hospital A and need immediate help.

• If the doctor has no attending privileges, ask why. Some

able men and women have chosen to confine themselves strictly to office practice. They use the time other doctors spend commuting between offices and hospitals and serving on hospital committees for seeing extra patients. When they hospitalize a patient, they make arrangements through someone with the appropriate skills. They're not second-class doctors by any means, but you'll have to decide for yourself whether that necessity of a referral for hospitalization is a detraction.

Hospital size

• **Large hospitals.** Not every community has a university hospital center, but many have large hospitals (with 250 beds or more) or medical centers. These large hospitals are more likely to have specialized equipment, coronary and intensive-care units, and the like. Also, the more restricted the staff privileges, the more likely it is that peer review will keep marginal practitioners off the staff.

• **Medium-sized hospitals** with 100 to 250 beds are called community hospitals. They are often "non-profit associations" that have been in operation for 25 or more years. Often they were started by churches and some still maintain the affiliation in their name ("Lutheran Hospital," "Methodist Hospital," and so on). Despite such links, most are non-denominational and have broad-based community support. They have good standards and screen applicants who want staff privileges.

• **Small hospitals** may be "for profit" or proprietary (owned by one or more physicians, sometimes even called "Doctors' Hospital"). The physician-owners may be very good doctors, but their standards are generally not as high as those of community hospitals. Other such hospitals are owned by companies and are part of a corporation. Controls are often looser, and peer review is not as strict as it is in larger hospitals.

Family physicians

A decade ago, the family doctor was a vanishing breed. Today, thanks to the determined efforts of the American Academy of Family Practice (A.A.F.P.), more young doctors are preferring this specialty to surgical and other specialties.

• **The new family physician is intensely trained.** Three years of residency with active, supervised patient-care training in obstetrics, pediatrics, minor surgery and psychotherapy are now required. Family doctors can now deal with more of your problems and refer you prudently when you need other specialized skills. Hospital affiliations (once denied) are no longer a problem either.

• **The practicing family physician must continue learning as well.** In order to remain board-certified, the doctor must pass an exam every six years. These specialists can't loaf— they must take seminars and post-graduate courses throughout their practice.

Medical Credentials

The credentials "game" is getting to be quite complicated these days, so a few notes about it are important.

1. **Residency.** After a physician is awarded an M.D. degree, there is a post-graduate specialty training period called a residency. The residency program will vary from two to five years—usually three.

2. **Board eligibility.** At the end of that time, the physician goes into medical practice and in two to five years takes the specialty board exams (a written and oral testing of skills and knowledge). When the test is successfully passed, the physician becomes certified by the specialty group.

3. **Specialization.** A surgeon then becomes a Fellow, American College of Surgeons, and will list after his name John Jones, M.D., F.A.C.S. A specialist in internal medicine becomes Fred Finley, M.D., F.A.C.P. (Fellow, American College of Physicians).

Other primary-care practitioners

In addition to family doctors, other physicians are also trained to serve as principal health-care managers.

• **Pediatricians, internists and obstetrician-gynecologists,** while trained as specialists in their fields, are interested in your general health and can serve as health-care partners. They can do an excellent job of coordinating your care, making referrals and so on.

• **Nurse-practitioners and other paraprofessionals** generally can't do some things physicians can do, like admitting you to a hospital, performing surgery or prescribing some drugs. (In some states, however, nurse-practitioners are licensed to practice independently.) However, they can be your primary contact with the health-care system, seeing you for your regular care and preventive treatment. Similarly, physicians' assistants and paramedics greatly extend the care a single physician can provide you, and are plusses in any medical practice you consider.

• **The disadvantage** in working with these primary-care practitioners, rather than with a family physician, is that your whole family may not be able to "qualify" for treatment by a single person. Thus you may wind up with a pediatrician for your children and an obstetrician-gynecologist or internist for adults in your family. Family physicians can treat everyone, and thus are able to note congenital, hereditary or environmental factors as part of their in-depth acquaintance with your family and its medical history.

Allied health professionals

There are several new health workers in the medical world that you will find offering primary care services: nurse-practitioners, pediatric nurse-practitioners, physicians' assistants (P.A.s) and paramedics. All have had special training to equip them for their duties. All perform regular clinical duties and some provide special surgical services.

• **The nurse-practitioner** is a nurse with an extra year or two of training that focuses on diagnostic testing, history taking and medical record-keeping.

• **The physician's assistant** has basic medical/nursing training and can assist with routine history taking.

• **The paramedic** often has previous military medical training and is specially prepared for emergency care (often paramedics are part of rescue squads and ambulance teams).

Professional affiliations

• **Medical V.I.P.s.** If your health-care partner-to-be is pres-

ident of the hospital staff or county medical society, that suggests that he or she *probably* has a higher than average sense of civic responsibility and humanitarianism. That's a good sign of the quality of patient care. Such people have earned the respect of their colleagues, too. However, your doctor can't do your gallstone in Lincoln, Nebraska, much good from the podium of an AMA convention in Las Vegas—so beware of professional joiners or medical politicos.

• **Professional societies.** Every physician should belong to three or four of these societies. Medical knowledge is expanding at an awesome rate, so special-interest society mem-

Pros and Cons for Different Medical Practices

There are exceptions to every rule, but the advantages and disadvantages of various kinds of medical practices are widely acknowledged. Combine the information below with the other data you accumulate as you search for a health-care professional, and you'll make the best choice.

Type of Practice	Pros	Cons
Solo: single physicians with self-contained staffs, equipment.	• Always the same doctor. • Attracts independent types. • Dedicated, personal care.	• May not be exposed to newest techniques, knowledge. • Little formal evaluation of medical practices. • Frequently overworked. • Coverage may suffer on "off" hours, vacations. • Less capital for equipment, facilities.

(continued)

Pros and Cons for Different Medical Practices *(continued)*

Type of Practice	Pros	Cons
Combined solo: individual physicians sharing staff, facilities by virtue of having adjacent offices.	• Lower overhead than with solo; more money for equipment, staff. • Supplemental coverage for "off" hours. • Informal contact for testing opinions.	• Same as solo (see above), but with better prospects for equipment, staffing.
Group/single specialty: physicians pooling staff, facilities, equipment and patient coverage in a clinic setting.	• Ability to hire and use more medical and clerical support staff. • On-the-spot conferencing, informal testing of opinions, education. • Continuous patient coverage. • Group screens new physicians so quality care is assured.	• Loss of personal touch. • Problems outside the specialty must be referred outside.
Group/multiple specialty: physicians with diverse specialties pooling staff, facilities, equipment and patient coverage in a clinic setting.	• Full range of services available. • In-clinic referrals when necessary. • On-the-spot conferencing, informal testing of opinions, education. • Continuous patient coverage. • Group screens new physicians so quality care is assured.	• Loss of personal touch if single health-care manager isn't used, but well-managed clinics overcome this with efficient use of allied professionals and patient advocates.
Health Maintenance Organization (HMO): group practice with multiple specialties (see above).	• Prepaid fee includes screening, preventive care, expensive emergencies. • Medications available at cost.	• Loss of personal touch if single health-care manager isn't used.

berships are essential if professionals are to have access to the meetings and journals that are important. There are groups for every disease and situation, dealing with muscular dystrophy, cancer, psychotherapy, computer medicine — the list goes on and on.

Medical records

You can judge something about a health-care professional by the records he or she keeps.

• **The best record system starts with your first visit.** Ideally your doctor should take a thorough baseline history — not just a cursory yes-no questionnaire, but one that really jogs your memory of symptoms, problems and lifestyle. Probing follow-up questions (with notes of your answers) should be part of it.

• **The worst systems are not systematic.** Collections of index cards, scrambled chronology in reports for visits, missing lab-test reports, and so on are symptoms of poor organization, which might obscure important patterns in your health picture.

• **Your access to medical records about yourself is guaranteed by law.** Many states have a "Patient's Bill of Rights" regarding your medical records. If your doctor or health professional refuses a serious request for review of your own records, you may have legal recourse. It is best, however, to seek health care from professionals whose trust and honesty with you make these legalistic demands unnecessary. The best care will come

from a relationship based on mutual respect.

• **Many fine doctors** discourage patient reviews of their own records, feeling that this places undue burdens on their patients to interpret technical data about themselves. The best arrangement is one that's mutually satisfactory, so discuss this with your doctor as you get acquainted.

Prescription practices

Apart from inquiring about your prospective health-care partner's attitudes about drugs that have significance for you, you need to know about his or her general practices with prescriptions and routine lab work like urine and throat cultures.

• **Ask about generic drugs** as options in prescriptions (they may save you money). Find out about the doctor's feelings about over-the-counter drugs as well. And does he or she make a practice of giving patients literature on drugs' side effects, the best ways to administer drugs, and so on?

• **Ask about cultures** (for throat or urinary infections) without full-dress office calls. If you can get these, you can save a lot of money and take advantage of important screening tests for serious diseases (see pages 136 and 161).

• **Ask about a pharmacist** the doctor recommends. A knowledgeable pharmacist can continue the job your doctor begins with helpful information and record-keeping for you.

Patient advocacy and education

Your prospective health-care partner's attitude about your involvement in your own health care is important. In addition to his or her personal style and receptivity to your involvement, you can ask about his or her support for patient education. Ask too about your hospital's use of patient advocates.

• **Patient advocates,** sometimes called ombudsmen, act on behalf of patients when their rights are in question. They may be involved in helping patients locate records, contact a chaplain or lawyer, arrange for financing or child care.

• **Patient educators** may be physicians, nurse-practitioners, nurses, paramedics or laypeople. They teach, one-to-one and in seminar or class settings, such topics as child care, cancer treatment, diabetes and other chronic problems, smoking cessation, weight loss and mutual support (for alcoholics, postmastectomy patients, members of families dealing with terminal illness), and so on.

Entering the Health-Care System

If you or a member of your family needs care today, what can you expect as far as care and costs go in the average-sized city? In order to give you an idea of what to expect, given the kind of health problem you have, look at page 86.

Primary care

• **On a typical day,** 80% of the individuals who enter the medical-care system (shown within the triangle on page 86) require *primary care*. This is care provided in the offices and clinics of family doctors, pediatricians, general internists and obstetrician-gynecologists.

• **The average person** needs such care about five times a year, and pays an average of $25 a visit.

Secondary care

• **If the problem requires hospital care** (delivering a baby, getting a broken leg set, having your gall bladder removed), the odds are you will have to go in only once in ten years.

• **The average cost** for that kind of care was $1,500 in 1980.

Tertiary care

• **More complex problems** (a rare blood disorder, cancer or heart disease requiring extensive surgery or treatment) fortunately occur on the average only once in 70 years—or once in a lifetime. These problems are expensive; costs averaged over $5,000 in 1980. This is the kind of problem described by the insurance people as "catastrophic."

Considering an HMO

If you have the option of joining an HMO (Health Maintenance Organization), ask yourself these questions to help judge

The Health-Care System

What are your odds of needing various types of health care?
The pyramid below shows how many people are served (and
at what cost) by the three major levels of the health-care
system in the United States. The average American thus may
spend $125 a year on routine care, $1,500 every decade on
hospital-related health care, and—once in a lifetime—$5,000
on a major health crisis.

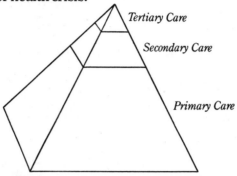

Tertiary Care
(surgical diagnostics
and treatment)
• **Average cost per incident:** $5,000
• **Frequency of incidents:** 1 per 70 years
• **Percentage of population affected:** 5%
• **Services:** cancer therapy, hip replacements, coronary
                  bypasses, pacemaker implantations

Secondary Care
(surgical specialties)
• **Average cost per incident:** $1,500
• **Frequency of incidents:** 1 per 10 years
• **Percentage of population affected:** 15%
• **Services:** labor and delivery, appendectomy,
                  set fractures, hernia repair, gall-bladder removal

Primary Care
(family physicians, ob-gyns,
pediatricians, internists)
• **Average cost per incident:** $25
• **Frequency of incidents:** 5 per year
• **Percentage of population affected:** 80%
• **Services:** stitches, shots, lab tests,
                  routine office visits

whether it will be a good deal for you as a consumer.

• **Cost.** Is the monthly fee for you and your family (probably $100 to $115) likely to be more or less than you'll pay for health care otherwise? The average person pays about $125 for a year of health-care services, barring serious illnesses and accidents. You'll have to weigh the relative costs and risks based on your family's health and accident records.

• **Benefit packages.** Will your employer or group pick up part of your monthly fee? If so, figure that savings into your costs.

• **HMO terms.** Is the plan comprehensive? Does it offer prescription drugs at cost, cover complications and extended illnesses, include dental care?

• **Staff.** Will you have a chance to work with a specific professional and thus establish a pattern of familiarity and trust, or will you be served on a strict rotation basis?

Using the Cheapest Service

It's obvious that no matter what your arrangements are for health care, the less specialized the solution to your problem, the more money you'll save. Consider these cost-cutting guidelines.

• **Use the phone** to avoid an office visit whenever possible.

HMO Facts

Economists point out that since 40% of national health costs are related to hospital expenses, one way to save part of the health-care dollar is to keep people out of the hospital. This has been one of the factors behind the federal efforts to establish Health Maintenance Organizations (HMOs) over the last ten years.

Studies have shown that when enough of the population (about 10%) gets its care from HMOs, competition with the traditional fee-for-service doctors in the marketplace contains—or even lowers—some costs. Once this market penetration is reached, there is also competition in efficiency and type of services delivered.

• **Most states now have HMOs,** and several states like California, Minnesota, Wisconsin, Massachusetts, New York, Washington and Oregon have organizations in most of their major cities. Corporations with large numbers of employees have been especially interested in helping get HMOs started.

• **There has been limited acceptance** by doctors and hospitals in most states, however.

• **Payment for HMO service** is based on a flat, fixed monthly fee for all care *paid before the service is provided.* Typically this is $80 to $100 per family, per month.

- **Look into convalescent homes** as alternatives to costly hospital stays.

- **Finally,** use ambulances and emergency rooms *only* when you're faced with a really serious problem—and nothing else will do.

Health care resources
- Ronald Gotts and Arthur Kaufman, *The People's Hospital Book* (Crown Publishers, 1978).

- S. Isenberg and L. M. Elting, *The Consumer's Guide to Successful Surgery* (St. Martins Press, 1976).

12 Ways to Cut Health-Care Costs

1. When you receive medical service, don't be reluctant to ask the doctor for a discount if you pay on the spot. This saves some billing costs.

2. Select a doctor to be "your doctor." Set up a relationship with the physician. Ask questions about costs. Ask for referrals if needed. Don't try to do your own "shopping" for specialists—often an expensive undertaking.

3. Use the telephone. Most doctors don't charge for telephone advice. Describe your symptoms after checking the self-care guide in this book. (See page 117.)

4. When it's not an emergency, go to the doctor's office, not the hospital's E.R., which will cost two or three times more than an office call.

5. If you are going to a hospital for surgery, inquire about "pre-admission testing." Such service provides for having the necessary lab tests done before you are admitted. Every day cut off the stay can save a bundle.

6. Ask if your surgery can be done on a one-day, come-and-go basis. If not, find out the earliest date you can get out of the hospital.

7. While in the hospital you have the right to ask the doctor why a certain test or procedure is being done—and what it costs.

8. Join a blood donor program *before* you need blood.

9. Don't pester your doctor to give you a prescription. Many drugs such as antibiotics and tranquilizers are overprescribed because patients feel they need one. If you do need one, ask for a proven, reliable generic form (rather than a brand name); it may be 50% less expensive.

10. Keep good records about drug and medical expenses so you can file for credit on your income tax.

11. Take a medical self-care course. You should be able to cut $100 to $200 a year from your medical bills when you can handle routine ailments and common injuries yourself.

12. Don't hesitate to request a second opinion if you're faced with a serious health problem. The added expense may only confirm some unpleasant news, but it could lead to alternative treatments or shed light on a confusing situation.

Chapter 8

Self-Care: Taking Charge of Your Health

When I was on the faculty of Georgetown University, I taught medical self-care skills to a group of sixth-graders in order to help them learn how to handle common injuries and ailments. I also wanted to find out what their attitude was toward taking charge of their own health.

At the start of the course, I asked the students to name and rank the people who play the most important roles in keeping them healthy. They ranked their doctors first, followed by the office nurses, their mothers, their fathers and finally, themselves.

These kids believed what the grownups around them believed: they could live however they wanted, eat as much as they wanted, smoke as much as they wanted, drink as much as they wanted—and then, if they got into trouble with their health, a doctor would bail them out. The bail-out would be accomplished with the help of the hospital, laboratory and drugstore.

By the end of the sixth-graders' course, an important change in belief had occurred. The students now ranked themselves as *most* important and their doctors as *least* important in determining their own health

status! They had learned what thousands of Americans are discovering—that individuals can and must be in charge of their own health affairs most of the time.

In doing so, they move from the traditional, passive patient's role to an active one. And doctors are recognizing the wisdom of Dr. Albert Schweitzer, who told physicians, "Each patient carries his own doctor inside him. They come to us knowing *that truth*. We are all at our best when we give the doctor within each patient a chance to go to work."

New Roles for Patients

Lay medical courses that were considered avant-garde in the early 70s—teaching people how to take their own blood pressures and pulses, to record their own symptoms and to learn home treatments for the common ills—are commonplace in most major cities now. The self-care education movement is picking up speed despite the fact that 96¢ of every health-care dollar still goes for diagnosis and treatment, leaving very little for education.

Even major corporations are beginning to recognize the need for self-care education for their employees. As these corporations develop health promotion programs as part of their employee benefit packages, health insurance companies may be forced to pay more and more for educational services.

Doctors, nurses, nurse-practitioners, physicians' assistants, dentists, pharmacists and health educators—not to mention patients—are getting a number of benefits from such education:

• improved doctor-patient relationships and care

• greater professional satisfaction

• prospects of fewer malpractice suits

• improved use of services (fewer unnecessary phone calls, better reporting of symptoms and so on)

• real financial benefits and reduced health care costs

So it's no wonder that there is widespread support for patients taking an active role in their health care. This section will tell you how to start taking a *more* active role in managing your health. Begin now, before a health crisis calls for urgent action!

Creating a good health-care team

It will be difficult to take charge of your health if the people who assist *you*—your physician, nurse-practitioner, dentist, pharmacist—don't endorse and support your efforts. The tips in Chapter 7 will help you locate a team that will welcome your active participation. Here are some additional suggestions for how to use your team.

• **Consider your complete team as you line it up.** Ideally, your physician (or other professional) will have or know of resources such as literature, classes and the like to boost your medical know-how.

• **Find a good pharmacist,** one who will continue to help in educating you, keeping good medication records for you and giving you good consumer information.

• **Evaluate the hospital you'd be referred to** for its in- or outpatient care. If you find its policies don't encourage patient rights and education, register your complaints with its administrators or your state's hospital licensing board. Laypeople are gaining increasing stature in forming policies, so use your clout to shape the system to suit your best interests.

Getting educated

• **Find out what's offered for self-care education** in your community. Your medical team should know of many options. Municipal, county and state organizations, as well as medical schools and university health services, support teaching programs too. And if you work for a forward-thinking firm, you may find on-site programs and services are available.

• **Take a medical self-care course.** After only eight to ten evenings of casual but practical classes, you can improve your ability to manage your health and cut health-care costs through prevention of and informed responses to problems.

Getting equipped

• **Go shopping** for the basic health-care and emergency supplies listed on page 119.

Knowing Whom to Call

Each time you deal with a health problem, you need to know whose help (if any) you need.

These guidelines will help you evaluate any situation. But remember that the key to evaluating things well is being an informed consumer. With good self-care knowledge, you can determine the best course of action.

Call an ambulance or rescue squad

• Only if the problem you're facing is life-threatening, or the patient needs hospital care and simply can't get there by car. A car will get you to a hospital faster anyway, as a rule, because it's only a one-way trip!

• Many municipalities charge you for ambulance runs (you could expect a $150 charge for a short run, which may or may not be covered by your insurance policy).

• Some rescue squads will refer you to a private ambulance company if you're not really facing a life-threatening situation. (See page 126 for definitions of serious medical emergencies.)

Call the doctor's office after hours

• When you need additional advice: whether to go directly to the hospital emergency room, whether to wait until the morning (or until Monday) to get treatment, whether a condition you're being treated for has taken a bad turn that requires immediate attention.

• Many large private clinics and HMOs staff their off-hour phones with nurses who are specially trained to dispense self-care information and gather your questions and symptoms, so the physician who returns your call can be well-informed when he or she calls back.

(continued)

Knowing Whom to Call *(continued)*

Call the doctor's office during regular hours

• When you need to schedule routine preventive care; when you need to ask if a problem warrants an office visit (and if not, to get instructions for home treatment); when you have to get results on lab work.

• With a good self-care education, you should be able to treat many ailments at home with just a call to confirm your proposed course of action.

• Much of this kind of contact needn't involve your physician if there is a good nurse-practitioner, office nurse or physician's assistant on hand.

• **Get the equipment** you'll need to take the readings of vital signs and make observations (see page 119-120).

• **If you have children,** examine your childproofing arrangements for medical supplies (see page 70).

• **Set up your own medical records.** The forms in this chapter can be duplicated and filled in, and then filed in a special place where they're handy when you need them. It will take only moments to keep them up-to-date; the information they contain is valuable in managing your own health.

Developing Your Health History

Your current health picture is a composite image of three factors: your inherited characteristics, your life's activities and the environment where you live, and finally, the events and situations that may create problems or change minor problems into major ones. If you keep a medical history of your family's health data, you can highlight (for yourself and your health-care team) the significant influences and patterns that affect you.

How to use these forms

• **Cut out or duplicate the forms** on the following pages (make copies for family members where applicable).

• **Fill in the information** requested on the forms as fully as possible. It may be necessary to contact family members and former physicians to get some of the information, but once you've gathered it, you'll have it permanently recorded.

• **Use the forms** when you contact a physician about a specific problem or when you get your periodic check-up. And post a copy of the Emergency Telephone Numbers Form near every phone in your house.

Emergency Telephone Numbers

_____
name of family member   date of birth   patient file number

_____
name of family member   date of birth   patient file number

_____
address (include directions for finding house if it's not easy to find, so emergency vehicles can arrive promptly)

Fire _____

Police _____

Rescue squad _____

Emergency room at hospital _____

Poison control center _____

Family doctors _____
                name family member(s) seen   office phone home phone

                   _____
                name family member(s) seen   office phone home phone

Dentist _____
          name   office phone   home phone

Pharmacy _____
            name   phone

24-hour pharmacy _____
                     name   phone

Father's work phone _____ Mother's work phone _____

Person to contact
in emergency _____
          name   address   phone

Taxi _____

Gas company _____

Electric company _____

Oil company _____

Water company _____

Other numbers _____

          _____

Emergency Consent Form

If your minor-aged child needs emergency medical care and you
aren't available to give your formal consent, the care may be
delayed—with serious, even fatal, consequences. Leave an
up-to-date Emergency Consent Form with your Emergency
Telephone Numbers list each time you leave a child with a
babysitter, and call the sitter's attention to it. The sitter will
need to bring it to the hospital if emergency care is necessary.
The form below is satisfactory.

To whom it may concern: In the event of any medical
emergency I/we hereby give my/our consent to Dr. _____
or whoever he/she designates to care for our child/children

_____ .
name(s)

_____
signature

_____
relationship   date

Address and directions to emergency room:

_____

_____

_____

_____

_____

Family History

Family Members (blood relations)	Type of Work	Lifestyle	
		Work-Related Hazards/Pathogens (DDT, mercury, etc.)	Stressful Events or Conditions (business, family problems, military duties, chemical dependencies, etc.)
Grandparents			
Parents			
Siblings			
Children			

Disease History

Check pertinent boxes to record
family members' health problems.

Family Members (blood relations)	Allergies	Diabetes	Drug abuse (incl. alcoholism)	Emotional Problem(s)	Heart Problem(s)	Hypertension
Grandparents						
Parents						
Siblings						
Children						

Disease History *(continued)*

Family Members (blood relations)	Stroke	Ulcers	Other	If Deceased, Age at Death	Cause of Death
Grandparents					
_____					
_____					
_____					
Parents					
_____					
_____					
_____					
Siblings					
_____					
_____					
_____					
Children					
_____					
_____					
_____					
_____					

Birth Records

Name	Date of Birth	Weight at Birth	Length at Birth	Delivery (normal/abnormal)	Condition at Birth	Feeding Method (breast/bottle)	Blood Type/Rh
Mother							
Father							
Children 1.							
2.							
3.							
4.							
5.							

Immunizations and Diseases Chart

Names		Father	Mother	Children		
		Date or Imm.	Date or Imm.	Date or Imm.	Date or Imm.	Date or Imm.
Diptheria	*First*					
	Second					
	Third					
Tetanus	*Boosters*					
Whooping Cough						
Polio	*First*					
	Second					
	Third					
	Booster					
Rubella						
Measles						
Mumps						
Chickenpox						
Hepatitis						
Strep Throat						
Scarlet Fever						
Rheumatic Fever						
Tuberculosis (note tests for)						
Other:						

Medications History

Date	Family Member	Problem	Medication Used (incl. strength of dosage)	Result/ Comment	Allergic Reaction?

Lab Report Record

A record of your lab test results will cut out unnecessary duplications and give you a personal health file similar to the one your physician keeps.

Family Member	_____
Date	_____

Blood Count (CBC)
   Hemoglobin _____
   Hematocrit
   WBC _____
   Differential _____
   RBC _____
   Sed. rate

Family Member	_____
Date	_____

Blood Chemistry
   Glucose _____
   Triglycerides _____
   Cholesterol _____
   Uric acid _____
   Other (list)

Family Member	_____
Date	_____

Urinalysis

Family Member	_____
Date	_____

Electrocardiogram
(EKG)

Family Member	_____
Date	_____

X-Ray (type)

Family Member	_____
Date	_____

Pap Test

Family Member	_____
Date	_____

Other

Important Medical Events Record

Family Member	Date	Age	What Happened (including complications)	Physician

Dental Record

Family Member	Date	Age	What Happened (including complications)	Dentist

Directory of Family Members' Doctors

Use this directory to record information about all the doctors your family goes to. Keep changes up-to-date so medical records can be located and referred to quickly.

Family Member	Doctor's Name, Address and Phone Number	Type of Doctor	Date Started with Doctor	Date Ended with Doctor
1.				
2.				
3.				
4.				
5.				
6.				
7.				
8.				

Recording Symptoms and Vital Signs

Once you have your family history and medical records set up, you should be in fine shape to respond to the inevitable health problems that will arise. To do so, you should be attuned to the language your body uses to speak to you in both sickness and health (much as you are attuned to the sounds of your car). You should also be able to measure and record both your normal and abnormal vital signs (temperature, pulse, respiration rate, blood pressure). Records of these vital signs will help you and your health-care team diagnose and treat your problems.

Listening to body talk

An important part of your own health care is to learn the language of symptoms as indicators of what is wrong with you. Ask yourself two basic questions when you notice any kind of symptom.

• **When does it occur?** Make mental notes about the why, when, where and what. Ask yourself if the symptom follows any pattern: does the backache always come after you've been sitting in a certain chair or car? Does the indigestion always follow your morning coffee? Is the symptom tied to any other symptoms?

• **Does it have a minor cause,** one you can deal with yourself? If it is unusual, severe or persistent, or if you are in any doubt about your conclusions, check it out with a professional. Your answers about when the symptom occurs will help your health-care partner move more quickly to a diagnosis.

Taking your temperature

Your temperature is a measure of the balance between heat production and loss in your body. Exercise, shivering, muscle tension, infection and external warmth produce heat and make your temperature rise. Sweating, panting, fatigue and external cold draw heat away and lower your temperature.

The purpose of taking your body temperature is to determine if the balance of your heat production and loss is stable. In a healthy person, this would be an oral temperature of 98° F. (37° C.), though there are variations in "normal" temperatures. Several factors that affect temperatures are listed below.

• **Time of day.** Temperatures are lower in the morning, higher in the late afternoon.

• **Age.** Infants (older than three weeks) and children have a slightly higher normal reading.

• **Emotions.** When you get "hot under the collar," your body temperature is likely to rise in anticipation of action.

• **The site where the temperature is taken.** Rectal temperatures are routinely 1° higher than oral or axillary (armpit) temperatures.

• **Illness from infection.** The body kills germs with higher temperatures.

How to Take Temperatures

Oral temperature
Note: readings will be inaccurate if the person has had something to drink in the last 15 minutes.

1. Shake mercury level down to below 98.6°F. (37°C.).

2. Insert thermometer under person's tongue.

3. Ask the person to close mouth and breathe through nose.

4. Take thermometer out after three minutes.

5. Read highest level of mercury; record reading.

Rectal temperature
Note: temperatures from rectal readings will be 1° higher than others.

1. Shake mercury level down to below 98.6°F. (37°C.).

2. Lubricate bulb with vaseline jelly.

3. Insert the bulb and no more than 1½ inches of the stem into the person's anus.

4. Take thermometer out after two minutes.

5. Wipe off thermometer and read highest level of mercury; record reading.

Axillary (armpit) temperature
Note: this method is less accurate than the two methods above and is therefore less preferable.

Same method as oral procedure above, but place the bulb on the skin under the person's armpit and keep it in place for five minutes.

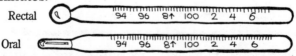

Rectal

Oral

Taking your pulse

Each time the heart pumps blood out of itself into the cardiovascular system, a pulse wave is generated (like the ripple that is generated on the water surface when you throw a stone into a pond). You can feel this pulse wave in places where your arteries come close to the surface of your skin.

The purpose of taking your pulse is to determine how fast your heart is beating (i.e., pumping). Common sites to take your pulse are at your wrist, forehead and the carotid area of your neck (near your jawbone). The usual rate is from 60-80 pulses a minute, though varia-

How to Take Pulses

Note: It is best to take your pulse while you are at rest, sitting in a comfortable position. You will need a watch with a second hand.

Wrist site

1. Lay your index and middle fingers across the inner surface of your wrist, about an inch from the base of your thumb.

2. Locate the pulse there (the radial artery pulse). Count the beats for 15 seconds, and multiply by 4 for the rate per minute.

Neck site

1. Tip your head to one side and tuck your index and middle fingers under the angle of your jawbone.

2. Straighten up your head and locate the pulse (the carotid artery pulse). Count the beats for 15 seconds, and multiply by 4 for the rate per minute.

Forehead site

1. Put your index and middle fingers along your hairline, about halfway between your ear and eyebrow.

2. Locate the pulse (the temporal artery pulse). Count the beats for 15 seconds, and multiply by 4 for the rate per minute.

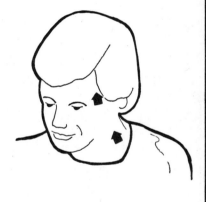

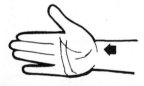

tions are caused by several factors, as listed below.

• **Age.** Children have higher pulse rates.

• **Exercise.** Your pulse speeds up after exertion as your heart pumps faster to meet increased demands for oxygen.

• **Emotions and pain.** Both raise your pulse.

• **Fever.** Your pulse will rise when you have a fever.

• **Time of day.** Pulses are slower in the morning and faster later in the day.

Taking your blood pressure

Blood pressure is the force your heart exerts on your blood to force it through the cardiovascular system in your body. The heart squeezes (contracts) and pushes blood through your veins and arteries to carry oxygen and

How to Take Blood Pressures

1. Have the person sit in a chair with the arm placed on a table or arm rest.

2. Wrap the cuff around the bare arm with the lower edge of the band at the crease where the elbow bends.

3. Place the head of the stethoscope under the cuff. Listen for heart sounds.

4. Inflate the cuff until the heart sounds disappear.

5. Slowly open the valve of the bulb of the sphygmomanometer until you hear the sounds again. Note the reading (e.g., 130).

6. Release the valve completely and let the air out of the balloon within the interior of the cuff. Note the reading when the heart sounds disappear (e.g., 80).

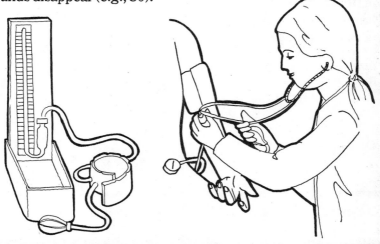

nutrients to (and wastes away from) all parts of your body.

Blood pressure is measured in terms of the millimeters of mercury it can push up when a cuff is wrapped tightly around a main artery. Using a cuff, you can measure both the systolic (heart contracted) and diastolic (heart relaxed) pressures. They are expressed as a ratio of systolic to diastolic pressure.

The normal range for systolic pressure is 100-145 millimeters of mercury; the normal range for diastolic pressure is 60-90. Several factors can influence your blood pressure.

- Emotional state related to stressful events in life
- Cigarette and smoking habits
- Amount of coffee (or caffeine-containing drinks such as tea, cola drinks) consumed each day
- Level of physical fitness
- Amount of salt used in food

How to Take Respiration Rates

The respiration rate is not as important as the other vital signs, but may provide useful information, particularly for asthma and emphysema victims. Here's how you determine it—it's very nearly impossible to take your own!

1. Ask person to sit upright or in a semi-upright position in a chair or bed.

2. Make sure that the normal breathing motion of the chest is not obscured with clothing or bedding.

3. Gently place the palm of your hand on the person's chest. (Put thumb in notch between collar bones on midline of chest.) Watch your hand move with each breath.

4. Count number of breaths in one minute. (Normal respiration rate is 12-14 breaths/minute.)

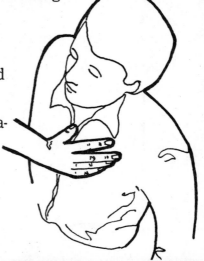

Taking your respiration rate

The rate at which you breathe helps to indicate how much oxygen you need—either how hungry your cells are for it or how efficiently you process it to get it to them. It's extremely variable, as you know from thinking about how slowly a person breathes when asleep compared to how fast a person pants after terrific exertion. These factors also affect respiration rates:

• Your emotional state (agitation, from good or bad causes, will speed respiration up)

• The presence of such conditions as asthma or chronic pulmonary disease, which decrease efficiency and raise the rate to compensate

• Smoking habits (smokers need to breathe more quickly because their lungs are less efficient)

• Level of physical fitness (lung efficiency increases with improved conditioning)

• The presence of a fever (the typical feverish child will breathe much more quickly than normally)

How to Do Breast Self-Examinations

It's important to examine your breasts following each monthly menstrual period (or on the first day of each month after menopause). Contact your physician if you notice any unusual lumps or dimples.

1. Lie down, placing your right hand beneath your head. With your left hand, gently push your fingers flat down on your right breast until you can feel the chest muscle.

2. For a reference point (in case you note a lump), mentally separate the breast into 4 clock-like sections: 12:00; 3:00, 6:00 and 9:00. Move your hand clockwise at 2-inch intervals, starting from 12 to 3. Continue making a circle from 3 to 6 and so on, until the entire breast has been covered.

3. Repeat the exam for your left breast using your right hand.

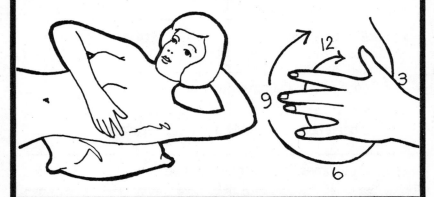

Making Office Calls Work

Armed with your history, medical records and symptoms, you are ready for an office call to get help with a medical problem. How can you get the best care?

• Avoid Mondays if possible. These are busy, catch-up-from-weekend days. Fridays are often busy too, as people suddenly foresee the weekend coming.

• Late afternoon (4 to 5 p.m.) is a poor time for an appointment. Schedules tend to be slipping then and the staff may be fatigued. (Mornings and early afternoons are *good* times.)

• If you are going to be late— or early—call ahead. The receptionist will appreciate the courtesy—and can help you.

• Plan to visit your doctor's office or clinic when you are well, and get a first-hand view of the facility.

How to Get the Most from an Office Call

This worksheet will help you get more from a visit to your doctor. Fill in the information as completely as you can.

Before Your Visit

1. Main reason for visit _____
2. Main symptoms (what, where, why) _____
_____
3. Medicines you are currently taking _____
_____
4. What you expect the doctor will do _____
_____
5. Additional matters or health concerns _____
_____
6. Insurance or health-care cards and forms to take _____
_____

During Your Visit

1. Name of the problem/condition
   (tentative? confirmed?) _____
2. Lab reports or diagnostic test results _____
3. Cause _____
4. Probable course of problem; time for recovery _____
_____
5. How to protect others from infection
   (if infectious) _____
6. Medication (if any; is a reliable
   generic form available?) _____
7. Side effects or notes on use of medication _____
_____
8. Ways to prevent recurrence of the problem _____
_____
9. Date to call for lab reports (if any) _____
10. Date of next visit (if needed) _____
11. Home care (diet, activity, treatment, precautions) _____
_____
12. Danger signs; reasons to call the office _____
_____

Smart Drug Use Checklist

The following checklist will help you to make the best use of the drugs you take. Remember to review this list before any visits to your doctor.

What to tell your doctor

☐ If you have had allergic reactions, such as rashes, headaches or dizziness, to drugs or foods you have taken in the past.

☐ If you are taking medicines or vitamins, including over-the-counter drugs and such special-category drugs as birth control pills or insulin, so the doctor will not prescribe a drug that could interact with one you're taking and cause unwanted side effects.

☐ If you are undergoing or have undergone medical treatment under the supervision of another physician.

☐ If you are pregnant or breastfeeding.

☐ If you have kidney or liver disease or any other special medical condition (such as diabetes).

☐ If you are on a special diet.

What to ask your doctor

☐ What is the name of the medicine? Write it down so you don't forget.

☐ What is the medicine supposed to do? (Relieve pain? Get to the cause of the pain? Reduce fever? Lower blood pressure? Cure infection?) How will you know it's working?

☐ What unwanted side effects might occur, such as sleepiness, swelling, nausea?

☐ Are there some medicines you should not take while taking this one? Some drugs cause reactions when taken with other drugs. (See pages 113-115.)

☐ How should you take the medicine? If you are told to take it "3 times a day," does that mean morning, noon and night? Should you take it before meals, with meals or after meals? If "every 6 hours," does that mean when you're awake, or should you get up during the night to take the medicine exactly every 6 hours?

☐ Are there any particular foods you should avoid while taking the medicine? Some antibiotics, for example, won't work if you drink milk or eat milk products. Alcoholic beverages should not be used when some drugs are being taken. (See page 113-115.)

(continued)

Smart Drug Use *(continued)*

☐ Should you take the medicine until it is all gone, or just until you feel better? Some medicines must be taken for long periods to cure the disease. If you stop the medication too early, even when you feel better, the symptoms and disease may recur.

How to get the most from prescription drugs

☐ If a drug is not doing for you what it is supposed to, check with your doctor. The doctor may wish to change the dosage or prescribe a different drug.

☐ After you start taking the drug, if you have an unexpected symptom—such as nausea, dizziness, headache and so on—report it to your doctor immediately.

☐ Read labels carefully for storing instructions. Some drugs should be kept cool and dry, others must be protected from light.

☐ Never let anyone else take medication prescribed for you, even if their symptoms seem to be the same as yours. The other person may be suffering from an entirely different problem—and certainly has a different medical history—so taking your medicine could be very dangerous.

☐ Do not transfer medicines from the containers in which they were dispensed. These containers are designed to keep the drug properly protected. Multipurpose pillboxes or other containers may not be suitable.

☐ Do not keep prescription drugs that are no longer needed. If you have medicines left over, destroy them.

How to Take Medications Carefully — and Safely

Take directly with, before or after meals

Aminophylline
APC
Artane
Aspirin
Azulfidine
Butazolidin
Cortisone Preparations
Darvon
DBI
Diabinese
Ferrous Gluconate
(don't take with antacids)
Ferrous Sulfate
(don't take with antacids)
Furadantin
Griseofulvin
Hycodan
Hycomine

Hydrocortisone
Hydrodiuril
Indocin
INH
Iron Preparations
(don't take with antacids)
Macrodantin
NegGram
Nydrazid
Orinase
PAS
Percodan
Prednisolone
Prednisone
Reserpine
Theophylline
Thiazide Preparations
Tolserol

Take on empty stomach (one hour before or two hours after meals)

Take with water only:

Ampicillin
Cloxacillin
Erythrocin
Erythromycin
Ilosone
Ledercillin VK

Nafcillan
Oxacillin
Penicillin G
Penicillin VK
Tegopen
Unipen

Take with water or fruit juice:

Achromycin*
Panmycin*
Sumycin*

Symycin*
Terramycin*
Tetracycline*

Take with plenty of water

Azo-Gantrisin**
Azulfidine
Gantrisin
Pyridium**
Succinylsulfathiazole

Sulfadiazine
Sulfapyridine
Sulfathalidine
Triple Sulfas

*Do not take these with milk or antacid preparations. One hour after taking medication, you can use milk/antacids.
**Unless directed otherwise by your physician, these medications should be taken ½ hour before meals. Urine may have an orange-red color from the medication.

(continued)

How to Take Medications Carefully— and Safely *(continued)*

Watch out for drowsiness and avoid alcohol or other depressants

Actifed	Librium
Ambrodryl	Lomotil
Atarax	Meprobamate
Benadryl	Miltown
Bonine	Ornade
Chlor-Trimeton	Phenergan
Codeine	Phenobarbital
Codeine Cough Syrup	Pyribenzamine
Cogentin	Serax
CoPyronil	Stelazine
Darvon	Teldrin
Demerol	Temaril
Dilaudid	Thorazine
Dramamine	Triaminic
Empirin Compound	Valium
Equagesic	Vistaril
Equanil	

Use no alcohol when taking

Amytal	Nitroglycerin
Antabuse	Noctec
BetaChlor	Noludar
Carbrital	Nydrazid
Chloral Hydrate	Orinase
DBI	Phenergan
Diabinese	Phenobarbital
Doriden	Placidyl
Dymelor	Quaalude
Elavil	Seconal
Flagyl	Somnos
INH	Thorazine
Insulin	Tolinase
M.A.O.I.	Tuinal
Nembutal	

Take with full glass of water, NOT mineral oil

Atropine Sulfate (take ½ hour before meals)	PeriColace
Belladonna Tincture (take ½ hour before meals)	Phenobarbital and Belladonna (take ½ hour before meals)
Colace	Pro-Banthine (take ½ hour before meals)
Metamucil	

(continued)

How to Take Medications Carefully— and Safely *(continued)*

Eat potassium-rich foods or take potassium supplements

Cortisone Preparations   Lasix
Edecrin   Prednisolone
Hydrocortisone   Prednisone
Hydrodiuril   Thiazide Preparations

To get the best from the above medications, one or more of the potassium foods below should be taken daily:

apricots   peaches
bananas   prunes
cantaloupe   raisins
orange and grapefruit juice

Discard after 10 days' use

Aureomycin Ointment
Chloromycetin Ophthalmic
Chloromycetin-Hydrocortisone Opthalmic

What's the Rx Mean?

Your doctor's handwriting ought to be illegible, according to tradition, but you may not be able to make sense of some of it even if you can decipher the letters. Here's a decoding chart.

SIG (signetur)—let it be labeled

PC (post cibum)—after meals

AC (ante cibum)—before meals

HS (hora somni)—at the hour of sleep (at bedtime)

QID (quater in die)—four times a day

TID (ter in die)—three times a day

Self-care resources

• Norman Cousins, *Anatomy of an Illness as Perceived by the Patient* (W. W. Norton, 1979).

• Arlene and Howard Eisenberg, *Alive and Well: Decisions in Health* (McGraw Hill Book Company, 1979).

• Timothy Rumsey and O. Otteson, *A Physician's Complete Guide to Medical Self-Care* (Rutledge Press, 1981).

• T. M. Roberts, K. M. Tinker and D. W. Kemper, *Healthwise Handbook* (Doubleday and Dolphin, 1979).

• Keith W. Sehnert with Howard Eisenberg, *How to Be Your Own Doctor (Sometimes)* (Grosset and Dunlap, 1975, 1981).

• Tom Ferguson, *Medical Self-Care: Access to Health Tools* (Summit Books, Simon and Schuster, 1980).

- D. M. Vickery and J. F. Fries, *Take Care of Yourself: A Consumer's Guide to Health Care* (Addison-Wesley, 1976).

- David S. Sobel, *Ways of Health* (Harcourt, Brace and Jovanovich, 1979).

Services

- American Medical Association
535 N. Dearborn
Chicago, IL 60010

- Health Activation Network
Box 923
Vienna, VA 22180

- Health Education Foundation
600 New Hampshire Ave. NW, Ste. 452
Washington, DC 20037

- National Center for Health Education
44 Montgomery St., Ste. 2564
San Francisco, CA 94104

- National Self-Help Clearinghouse
33 West 42nd St., Rm. 1227
New York, NY 10036

- National Women's Health Network
1302 18th St. NW, Ste. 203
Washington, DC 20036

Chapter 9

Illness and Emergency Guide

If this book had been written a decade or more ago, this chapter would have been called the "first aid" section, on the assumption that laypeople were only competent to provide stopgap assistance to the sick and injured . . . until the doctor could step in and take over. But in the last decade, health-care professionals have come to recognize that teamwork can benefit both sides: it can both ease professionals' work loads and give laypeople a sense of control over their own health, particularly when problems arise. This chapter is designed to give you the information you need to identify and respond to problems, whether or not you eventually need to involve a professional in your treatment.

How to Use This Chapter

Remember, this part of the book is not intended to replace professional help when that is necessary, but rather to help you decide when you need that help and when you don't—and to tell you what to do if you can handle the problem yourself. Please take time to read these preliminary pages carefully, and then familiarize yourself with the rest of the chapter. Doing so will give

you an advantage that may be crucial to you or others sometime in the future.

Features

You'll find a number of features here:

• **a list of supplies and health-care tools** that every home should have, plus ideas for storing them safely and a list of sources where you can get the more specialized items.

• **a how-to section for basic treatments,** like how to apply heat and cold, how to splint, bandage or wrap, and guidelines for calling for help immediately.

• **an explanation of the format** used in the remainder of this chapter.

• **an alphabetical list** of the entries in the guide.

• **a symptoms index** to the guide, so you can locate, for example, all the possible illnesses and injuries that could cause your runny nose or headache.

Health-Care Supplies

Having the right medications, emergency supplies and health-care tools on hand can make a big difference in your ability to prevent and respond to problems that may occur.

Medications and supplies

Your home medicine chest is the cornerstone of your self-care treatment program. The list below, in effect, will provide you with prescription and over-the-counter (OTC) medications and emergency supplies for most of the common ills you'll need to treat. Ask your physician to prescribe the ones you need his or her prescription for, with the understanding that you'll dispense them sensibly to yourself and your family, and call for advice if you notice complications in your self-treatment.

Medicine Chest Checklist

Name of Drug	Size Stock	Adult Dosage	Reason
☐Aspirin (also for children)	Many forms	1 or 2 tabs as needed	Pain, headache
☐Benadryl (also for children)	—	1 cap. every 4 hrs.; elixir as directed	Allergies
☐Debrox drops	½ oz.	5 drops daily	Ear wax
☐Di-Gel liquid	6 oz.	2 tsp. every 2 hrs.	Gas, acid indigestion
☐Emetrol	3 oz.	1-2 tsp. every hour	Nausea, vomiting
☐Hydrocortisone ointment	—	As directed	Itching skin
☐Lomotil	—	2 tabs, 3x daily	Diarrhea
☐Marezine tabs	24 tabs	1 tab as needed	Motion sickness
☐Neosporin ointment	½ oz.	2-4x daily	Abrasions, skin infections
☐Neosynephrine nose drops (also for children)	1 oz.	2-4 drops, 3x daily	Nasal congestion, sinusitis
☐Parepectolin	8 oz.	1-2 tbsp., 4x daily	Diarrhea
☐Robitussin syrup	4 oz.	As directed	Cough control
☐Tincture benzoin	1 oz.	As needed	Taping skin
☐Triaminic syrup	4 oz.	As directed	Colds, allergies
☐Tylenol (also for children)	Many forms	1 or 2 tabs as needed	Pain, headache

Emergency Supplies Checklist

- ☐ Absorbent cotton
- ☐ Activated charcoal (to absorb poison)
- ☐ Adhesive strip bandages, assorted sizes
- ☐ Adhesive tape, ½-1" wide
- ☐ Adolph's Meat Tenderizer
- ☐ Butterfly bandages
- ☐ Cotton-tipped swabs
- ☐ Drinking cups, paper or plastic
- ☐ Epsom salts (use only as directed by poison prevention center; also for soaking)
- ☐ Eye drops
- ☐ Household ammonia
- ☐ Hydrogen peroxide
- ☐ Insect sting kit (by prescription only, for allergic persons)
- ☐ Measuring cup
- ☐ Measuring spoons
- ☐ Merthiolate
- ☐ Penlight with fresh batteries
- ☐ Petroleum jelly
- ☐ Rubbing alcohol
- ☐ Safety pins
- ☐ Sharp needles (to remove splinters; sterilize first)
- ☐ Sharp scissors with rounded ends
- ☐ Snake bite kit (where appropriate)
- ☐ Sterile eye pads
- ☐ Sterile gauze bandages, assorted sizes, ½-2" wide
- ☐ Sterile gauze pads, 2" x 4"
- ☐ Syrup of ipecac (to induce vomiting)
- ☐ Thermometer (rectal for infants)
- ☐ Tongue depressors
- ☐ Triangular bandages, large
- ☐ Tweezers

Health-care tools

You may want to invest in a family black bag, which combines many of the tools you need for home medical care. Or you may want to assemble a black bag of your own. In either case, here are some invaluable tools, with information about their uses, costs and sources of supply.

• **Family black bag.** A complete kit of equipment, which includes a good quality otoscope, a stethoscope, a sphygmomanometer and a thermometer. Cost: complete kit—$120; kit without the otoscope—$78. Source: Marshall Electronics (Skokie, Ill.).

• **Stethoscope.** For checking heart sounds, chest congestion and breathing sounds; for taking blood pressures. Cost: $10 to $12. Sources: catalog companies such as Sears, Ward's and Penney's, many full-line department stores and most retail drugstores. Also can be part of family black bag (see above).

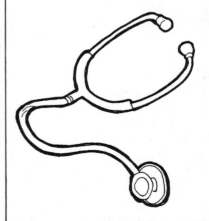

• **Sphygmomanometer.** For measuring blood pressures. Available as aneroid (dial) unit or electronic unit. Cost: aneroid unit—$27.50 to $45; electronic unit—$79 to $220. Sources: catalog companies such as Sears, Ward's and Penney's, many full-line department stores and most retail drugstores. Also can be part of family black bag (see page 119).

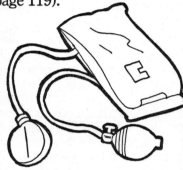

• **Otoscope.** For looking inside ears. Cost: $58. Source: Marshall Electronics. You can also put together your own inexpensive otoscope by buying a penlight at a drugstore or hardware store and pairing it with an ear speculum you can get from a surgical supply store for less than $2. It's not as satisfactory as a real otoscope, which magnifies the image and is more convenient to use.

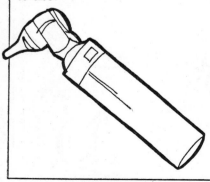

• **Thermometer.** For taking temperatures. Cost: under $2. Use a rectal thermometer for children; oral for adults. Source: any drugstore.

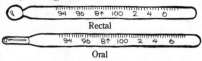

• **Penlight.** For examining throat, ears, nose. Cost: six for $1.90. Source: Marshall Electronics.

• **HotCold packs.** Packs that can be heated or chilled and applied as needed. Cost: about $4. Source: made by the 3M Company, available at most pharmacies.

Storing supplies

• **Keep medications, supplies and tools in a single area—**most likely you keep them now in your bathroom, but a drawer or linen chest is less exposed to moisture and heat (and is more childproof), and thus is preferable.

• **Store medications in a lockable cabinet** even if you don't have youngsters around routinely.

• **Near your supplies, post a list of key phone numbers** (see page 93). You should have them by your phone too, but keeping another set there wouldn't hurt.

Basic Treatments and Emergency Care

The following procedures will be required in your treatment of various problems, so they are presented here for ease of reference.

Applying Heat

The method you choose for applying heat should suit the part of the body you need to treat. Depending on the problem, you may need to apply moist or dry heat.

Treatment	Procedure
Hot compress for back, joints, limbs 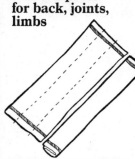	• **Wet a large towel** thoroughly in warm water; wring it out and fold in thirds lengthwise. Wrap it around or across the affected area. • **Repeat** twice daily. • **Other methods** are the new HotCold Packs available from 3M (see page 120) or a warm heating pad.
Hot compress for ears 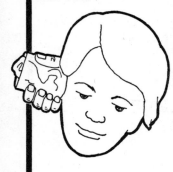	• **Soak paper towels** in hot water; wring dry. Stuff towels into a small, already-warmed water glass. • **Tilt affected ear** up and press bottom of glass over ear for 10 minutes. • **Rewarm glass and towels;** repeat for another 10 minutes. • **Or try a heating pad** or a hot water bottle.
Hot compress for eyes 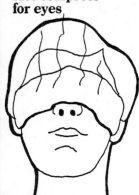	• **Soak a washcloth** or handkerchief in warm water; wring dry. (Don't use hot water, as it may cause tissue near the eye to swell.) • **Apply** once every 3 hours for 5 to 10 minutes. • **Try a cold compress** (same method but with cold water) if the eye is swollen or feels itchy. • **Add eye drops** after applying these compresses.

(continued)

Applying Heat *(continued)*

**Gargle
for throats**

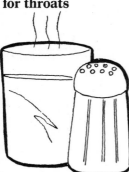

- **Make your own gargle solution:** add 1 tsp. of salt to 8 oz. of hot water.
- **Gargle** once every 2 hours for 5 minutes, until pain ends.
- **Or try a hot solution** of Cepacol or a similar product available at drugstores.

**Hot compress
for sinuses**

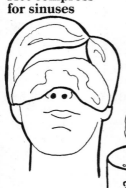

- **Soak one towel** in hot water; wring dry. Place on forehead or cheeks for 30 seconds.
- **Soak another towel** in cold water and ice cubes; wring dry. Place on forehead or cheeks for 30 seconds.
- **Alternate** these hot and cold compresses for 10 minutes.
- **Repeat** 4 times daily.

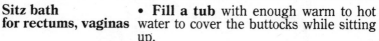

**Sitz bath
for rectums, vaginas**

- **Fill a tub** with enough warm to hot water to cover the buttocks while sitting up.
- **Sit** in this hot sitz bath for 10 to 15 minutes.

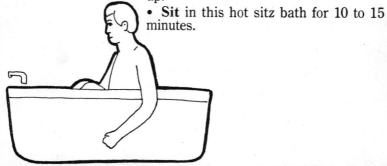

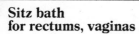

Applying Cold

There are several ways to apply cold to treat injuries and illnesses. Here are several basic procedures.

Treatment	Procedure
Cold compress to control bleeding 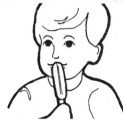	• **Apply** plastic bag filled with crushed ice to the affected area. • **Put a popsicle** on the cut if it's on a child's lip or cheek. The child will enjoy it —and there's no harm in swallowing a little blood!
Cold soak to treat injured ankles, arms, feet, hands, wrists	• **Immerse injured part** in bowl, styrofoam cooler or dishpan filled with cold water (with ice cubes if possible). Soak as needed.
Cold soak to lower fever	• **Immerse the person** in a tub half-full of tepid water. With a facecloth, drizzle water on back, face and chest; wet hair if practical. • **Avoid chilling** the person; 20 minutes should be sufficient to lower most fevers. • **A shower** can be substituted for the tub if necessary. • **If the patient can't be bathed,** place a plastic sheet or oil cloth under the person and apply cold towels that have been soaked in a solution of 2 quarts water, 1 pint rubbing alcohol and 1 quart ice cubes.
Cold compress to treat bruises, sinusitis, insect stings 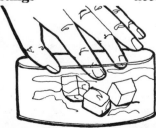	• **Put a dozen ice cubes** in pan with cold water; soak a towel in it. Wring towel dry and apply to the injured area. Repeat as needed.

Splints

Immobilizing an injured part of your body can allow it to heal more quickly in some cases. If you need to splint an extremity, these simple methods will help.

Fingers and toes

Tape fingers or toes to an adjacent finger or toe, with 2 or 3 pieces of ½"-wide tape.

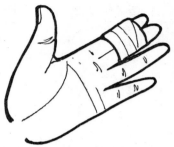

Wrist and forearm

Use a newspaper or magazine to immobilize the injured area, taping it or tying it with pieces of cloth.

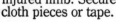

Leg

Take 2 boards or pieces of sturdy material and place them on either side of the injured limb. Secure them with cloth pieces or tape.

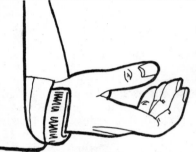

Ankle

Make a splint with towel or pillow, securing it with tape or pieces of cloth tied around the ankle area.

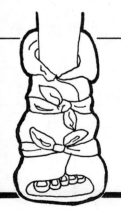

Bandages

Bandages keep dirt out of wounds and protect them from further injury. When they cover pads with medication or close cuts, they also promote healing.

Type	Procedure
Basic bandage	• **Clean** the affected area and control bleeding before applying the bandage. • **Use** a 2″ x 2″ or 4″ x 4″ sterile gauze dressing or an ouchless bandage (Telfa). • **Attach with adhesive tape** or roller gauze and tape.
Elastic bandage	• **Clean** area and apply dressings if needed. • **Begin wrapping** the area with even, gentle pressure. Do not bind the bandage too tightly! • **If you are directed to do so,** unwrap the bandage several times a day to relieve the pressure.
Butterfly closure 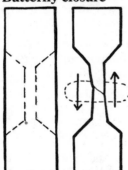	• **Use** a commercial butterfly closure or make one yourself using ½″ adhesive tape. • **Cut the tape** as shown; twist one end 360° until both ends have adhesive sides down. Then pull the edges of the wound together and apply. • **Cover** with a gauze bandage or Band-Aid (with a large wound you might need to wrap with an elastic gauze bandage).
Bandage removal 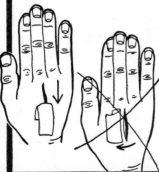	• **Once a bandage is in place,** it's best to leave it on for the first 24 hours. After that, remove and change bandages as often as necessary. • **Soak gauze** in cold water before removing to avoid disturbing the wound. • **Remove the bandage** lengthwise, as shown, to prevent the wound from reopening.

What's an Emergency?

We all recognize that there are emergencies and then there are *emergencies*. A bad fall might leave you with a number of aches and pains—and cause you a good deal of anxiety—but the odds are that you can respond to its effects with informed home care. The conditions below are different, however. If you note any of them, seek medical care *immediately.*

Unconsciousness	When you can't rouse someone, call for help.
Drowsiness (stupor)	When the person is conscious but unable to answer questions, get help. With children and infants, you may need to judge this in contrast with ordinary alertness.
Disorientation	When someone can't remember his or her name, the place or the date (in order of decreasing importance), get help. An injury or illness causing disorientation is serious.
Severe injury	You'll know it when you see it: large wounds, obvious bone fractures, extensive burns need more care than you can give.
Uncontrollable bleeding	Pressure should stop most bleeding; when it fails to, get help. Children can not afford to lose as much blood as adults can.
Shortness of breath	If a person is unusually short of breath even while resting, and you can rule out hyperventilation, which is most common in young adults (see page 142), get help.
Severe pain	While pain is subjective, and may be caused by emotional and psychological factors, a person in intense pain still needs relief from it. Don't take pain itself as a barometer of the seriousness of the emergency, but do seek relief from a professional.

How to Use the Guide

The following guide is designed to be self-contained and not require you to go to outside sources, but a few preliminary comments are necessary to help you use the guide most effectively.

Finding what you need

• **Flip through the guide,** glancing at the large-type headings at the top of the page. Chances are you'll locate the page you need in less than 10 seconds.

• **If you are unsure about what your problem is called,** check the symptoms index (see page 129). It will direct you to all probable listings.

• **See the sample entry** below to familiarize yourself with the format.

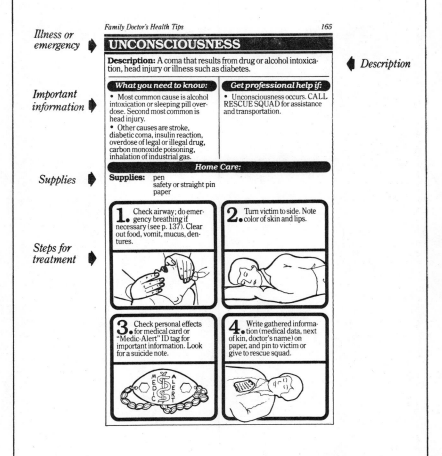

Illness or emergency ▶

Family Doctor's Health Tips   165

UNCONSCIOUSNESS

Description: A coma that results from drug or alcohol intoxication, head injury or illness such as diabetes.   ◀ *Description*

Important information ▶

What you need to know:	**Get professional help if:**
• Most common cause is alcohol intoxication or sleeping pill overdose. Second most common is head injury. • Other causes are stroke, diabetic coma, insulin reaction, overdose of legal or illegal drug, carbon monoxide poisoning, inhalation of industrial gas.	• Unconsciousness occurs. CALL RESCUE SQUAD for assistance and transportation.

Home Care:

Supplies ▶ **Supplies:** pen
safety or straight pin
paper

Steps for treatment ▶

1. Check airway; do emergency breathing if necessary (see p. 137). Clear out food, vomit, mucus, dentures.

2. Turn victim to side. Note color of skin and lips.

3. Check personal effects for medical card or "Medic-Alert" ID tag for important information. Look for a suicide note.

4. Write gathered information (medical data, next of kin, doctor's name) on paper, and pin to victim or give to rescue squad.

Illness and Emergency Guide Contents

Illness and Emergency Guide
Symptoms Index

ABDOMINAL PAIN

Description: Sensations of stretching, spasm or tearing in abdomen due to digestive, urogenital or cardiovascular problems.

What you need to know:

• There are two categories of abdominal pain: *acute* pain, which starts quickly and may require immediate action; and *chronic* pain, which recurs periodically in response to diet, emotions or disease.

• Sometimes the pain (*referred* pain) is felt in a part of the body that is distant from the actual site of the organ involved.

• This treatment plan is for common types of acute and chronic abdominal pain.

Get professional help if:

• Sudden, intense pain in abdomen, groin or back develops.

• A pattern of painful episodes involving those regions develops over time. Be prepared to describe the kind of pain, its location, its duration and the circumstances that bring it on (see below).

PAIN PATTERNS

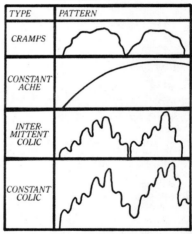

PAIN LOCATIONS
REFERRED
TO FRONT

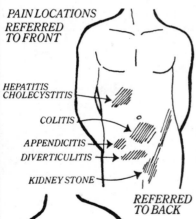

HEPATITIS
CHOLECYSTITIS

COLITIS

APPENDICITIS

DIVERTICULITIS

KIDNEY STONE

REFERRED
TO BACK

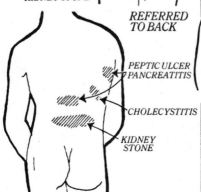

PEPTIC ULCER
PANCREATITIS

CHOLECYSTITIS

KIDNEY
STONE

PARTS OF YOUR
ABDOMEN

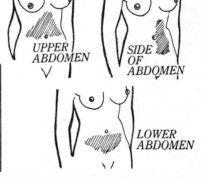

UPPER
ABDOMEN

SIDE
OF
ABDOMEN

LOWER
ABDOMEN

Home Care:

Supplies: thermometer   stethoscope
blood pressure unit   ice chips
watch with second hand

1. Symptoms:

Acute pain patterns

• **Appendicitis.** At first, pain is in upper abdomen near centerline (see p. 130). Later, pain may switch to lower abdomen on right. Pain pattern is gradual in onset and worsens over several hours, becoming a constant ache (see p. 130).

• **Cholecystitis** (gall bladder infection). Pain in upper abdomen on right or in back under right shoulder blade (see p. 130), usually after a fatty meal. Nausea and vomiting, followed by yellowing of skin and whites of eyes (jaundice), and dark urine, may occur.

• **Hepatitis** (yellow jaundice). Pain in upper abdomen on right, with pattern of dull, constant ache. Aching, fatigue, nausea, and yellowing of skin and whites of eyes may occur. Stool will be light color; urine will be dark brown.

• **Diverticulitis** (colon condition). Pain in lower abdomen on left, often occuring after cramping. Constipation, nausea, vomiting, rectal bleeding may occur.

• **Kidney stone.** Pain starts on side of abdomen and may be felt moving down into groin. Pattern of intense pain (constant colic), with cold sweating. Urinating may be painful, with blood.

• **Pancreatitis** (inflamed pancreas). Pain starts in upper abdomen, sometimes moving to back. Pattern is constant ache in mild to severe degree.

• **Salpingitis** (infection of the Fallopian tubes). Pain in lower abdomen, with severe intensity. Occasional vaginal discharge.

• **Ruptured ectopic pregnancy** (pregnancy in the Fallopian tubes). Sudden pain in lower abdomen, when last menstrual period more than 6 weeks past. Constant pain pattern.

Chronic pain patterns

• **Esophagitis** (reflux of acid back up from the stomach). Pain in upper abdomen at centerline or in jaws. Often occurs in obese people. Burning distress worsens while bending over or lying flat soon after meals.

• **Irritable colon.** Discomfort in lower abdomen. Pain pattern of cramps. Aggravated by anxiety and emotional upsets. Relieved by defecation or passage of gas.

• **Peptic ulcer.** Pain, distress (sometimes acute) in upper abdomen. Pattern is dull ache, 1–4 hours after meals. Worsens with alcohol, coffee, aspirin. Relieved by antacid or food.

• **Regional enteritis** (inflammation of small or large intestine). Pain in lower abdomen, often near navel. Soft, unformed stools. Weight loss common. Distress relieved by defecation.

• **Ulcerative colitis** (inflammation of large intestine). Distress in lower abdomen. Worsens before bowel movement. Recurring passing of small amounts of blood in stools. Weight loss common.

2. What to check:

• **Relation to eating.** Look for tendency for pain to occur 1–4 hours after meals, often occurring daily for several weeks (peptic ulcer). Check for distress 3–5 hours after meals, occurring only once or twice monthly (gall bladder disease).

• **Type of food.** Watch for pain after eating fatty foods such as butter, pork, salad dressings (gall bladder disease or cholecystitis). Look for distress after eating roughage—fresh vegetables and fruit (irritable colon or diverticulitis).

• **Physical position.** Look for pain that occurs when lying down at night (esophagitis), especially when distress is relieved by sitting up or getting up and walking.

3. Treatment:

For both acute and chronic pain

• Do NOT take laxative or enema.

• Limit all intake to ice chips or small sips of water at onset of pain.

• Assume whatever position is most comfortable; rest.

• Record pain patterns and other observations for use by health professional.

• Note temperature, pulse and blood pressure 3 times daily.

ALLERGIC STUFFY NOSE

Description: Inflammation and congestion of nasal passages caused by allergies to pollen, dust, food and other irritants.

What you need to know:

- 10% of population have some kind of nasal allergy each year.
- Minimizing dust and other irritants in rooms, making sure furnace is filtered, and checking to see that air conditioner is clean and working properly may prevent irritation.

Get professional help if:

- Symptoms increase over years and general preventive measures don't help.
- Mucus in nose is thick green or yellow.
- Antihistamines cause drowsiness and it's essential to drive or operate heavy machinery.

Home Care:

Supplies: penlight   nose drops
               antihistamines   glasses of water
               oral nasal decongestant

1. Symptoms:

- bloody nose
- congested nose
- coughing
- hoarseness
- itching eyes, nose
- red or watery eyes
- sneezing, runny nose
- trouble breathing

2. What to check:

- Have assistant examine nasal membranes with penlight. Pale, swollen, waterlogged (sometimes bluish) surface suggests allergy.
- Look for dark circles under child's eyes.
- Keep list of possible irritants.

3. Treatment:

- Take antihistamines or oral nasal decongestant several times a day for no more than 3 days. Then call doctor.
- Rest and stay indoors on windy days.
- Wash hands and face frequently on bad days or in allergy season.

- Use nose drops for relief at bedtime. LIMIT USE TO 3 TIMES A DAY FOR NO MORE THAN 3 DAYS.
- Drink one 8-oz. glass of water per hour to replace fluid lost in nasal discharge.
- Avoid alcohol (a congestant) and stop smoking (an irritant).

ARTHRITIS

Description: Stiffness and inflammation that usually affect the joints most used but can affect any joint.

What you need to know:

- This treatment plan is for common arthritis only.
- Other arthritic conditions are more crippling (rheumatoid arthritis; arthritis due to infection or gout; nonarticular rheumatism, called bursitis or fibrositis) and need professional help.

Get professional help if:

- Aspirin causes dizziness, ringing in ears, indigestion, pain in stomach or constipation.
- Pain is limited to 1 joint and there is family history of gout.
- General weakness or increasing fatigue develop.

Home Care:

Supplies: aspirin
                heating pad or hot water bottle
                ColdHot Pack (3M)

1. Symptoms:

- aching joints
- back, knee, hip pain
- bumps in and around joints
- dizziness, ringing in ear
- limping, trouble walking
- loss of appetite
- stiff wrist, shoulder, neck
- weather causes aching

2. What to check:

- Note time of day aching is worst.
- Note effect of aspirin.
- Examine fingers for knobby areas and bumps (Herberden's nodes) around joints.

3. Treatment:

- Apply heat (see p. 121).
- Take aspirin.
- Massage muscles *surrounding* joint (not joint itself) to improve circulation.
- Keep as active as possible to maintain muscle strength (swimming is especially good). If joints are painful, rest after activity.

- Wear extra clothing for warmth in cold weather.

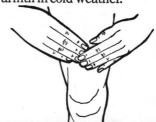

ASTHMA

Description: A lung condition associated with allergies. Linings of bronchial tubes are inflamed, swollen and clogged with mucus.

What you need to know:

- Asthma distress can be a frightening experience. Keeping calm may reduce the severity of the attack.
- Causes include smoke, dust, pollen, infection, food, medication, exertion, damp weather, emotional stress, fatigue.

Get professional help if:

- Individual can not talk, eat or lie flat in bed to sleep.
- Temperature over 101° several times in 1 day.
- Sputum changes from clear white to yellow, green, gray or red.
- Vomiting occurs more than twice in a few hours (especially children).

Home Care:

Supplies: thermometer asthma medication
stethoscope glasses of water
watch with second hand

1. Symptoms:

- aching in chest
- breathing pain, wheezing
- congested or runny nose
- coughing, hoarseness
- fever
- shortness of breath
- sleeping trouble
- sneezing

2. What to check:

- Note all possible irritants.
- Note temperature 3 times daily.
- Check breathing rate at rest (normal is 18–20 breaths/minute for adults).
- Check pulse rate at rest (normal is 68–72 beats/minute for adults).

3. Treatment:

- Follow suggested allergy prevention techniques (see page 133).
- Start asthma medication as soon as possible; continue until wheezing stops.
- DO NOT USE SPRAY FORMS OF ASTHMA MEDICATION WITHOUT MEDICAL ADVICE. They may worsen asthma.
- Drink one 8-oz. glass of water, juice or tea every hour.
- Avoid all known irritants.
- If child develops stomachaches from swallowing large amounts of mucus, help child to vomit.

BLADDER INFECTION

Description: An infection of the bladder and urethra that in some cases spreads up to ureters and kidneys.

What you need to know:

• Properly and promptly treated, this disease is self-limiting: it runs its course in 3 days.
• Usually caused by bacteria, but sometimes a virus is at fault.
• More common in women.

Get professional help if:

• Diabetic.
• History of kidney disease.
• Blood in urine (hematuria) persists for 24 hours.
• Pregnant.
• Symptoms persist after 24 hours of home treatment.

Home Care:

Supplies: thermometer
glasses of water
aspirin

1. Symptoms:

• back/lower abdominal pain
• bed wetting/night urination
• blood in urine
• burning urination
• change in odor, color of urine
• chills/fever; sweating
• frequent urination
• pain over pubic area

2. What to check:

• Note temperature 3 times daily.
• Punch kidney very gently on each side. Is there pain? If so, suspect kidney infection and call doctor (see p. 130).
• Record color of urine.

3. Treatment:

• Increase liquid intake to replace lost fluids; drink 8 oz. water or juice every hour.
• If feverish, rest in bed to conserve energy and shorten illness.
• Take aspirin for pain— especially useful at bedtime.

• Take hot sitz baths in tub (¼ filled with warm water) to relieve burning (see p. 122).
• Avoid alcohol, tea, coffee, which are urinary tract irritants.

BREATHING EMERGENCY

Description: Life-threatening condition that results from blocked airway or cardiac arrest.

What you need to know:

• The basic steps in a breathing emergency (the A–B–Cs of cardio-pulmonary resuscitation) are: **Airway→Breathing→Circulation.**

• Do not attempt neck lift with suspected neck fracture.

Get professional help if:

• Breathing, heart beat, and pulse do not resume after you follow the treatment below.

Home Care:

Supplies: syringe plastic airway

1. Place patient on back. Put your ear close to his mouth to detect breathing. Clean out mouth with syringe. Insert plastic airway.

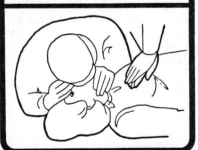

2. If patient is not breathing, raise neck with 1 hand; push forehead down with other hand. If patient does not start breathing, pinch nostrils shut and blow air into mouth. When chest moves up, take your mouth away and let chest go down. Do 4 quick full breaths without allowing time for patient's lungs to fully deflate. For infants and children, cover both mouth and nose with your mouth; use smaller breaths once every 3 seconds.

3. If cardiac arrest occurs, apply pressure rhythmically over lower half of chest plate. Alternate with emergency breathing.

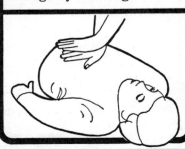

4. If there is 1 rescuer, perform both breathing and circulation with a 15 to 2 ratio (after 15 chest compressions at a rate of 80/minute, 2 very quick lung inflations). If 2 rescuers, perform both breathing and circulation with a 5 to 2 ratio (after 5 chest compressions at a rate of 60/minute, 2 lung inflations). For infants and children, do same with less force and faster compression rate (80 to 100/minute).

BRONCHIAL INFECTION

Description: Infection of the lower windpipe (bronchus) caused by bacteria or viruses.

What you need to know:

• Chronic bronchitis can lead to serious chronic obstructive lung disease, if untreated.
• Bronchitis is contagious; take precautions to isolate patient.

Get professional help if:

• History of chronic lung disease or bronchitis.
• Cough persists.
• Over 60 years old.
• Pulse over 100 beats/minute.
• Temperature over 101° several times in 1 day.
• Respiration rate over 25/minute.

Home Care:

Supplies: thermometer   glasses of water
stethoscope   cold air vaporizer
watch with second hand cough medicine

1. Symptoms:

• aches or chest pain (adults)
• bad breath
• chills/fever; sweating
• coughing or coughing up blood
• hoarseness; sore throat
• runny nose
• wheezing

2. What to check:

• Note temperature 3 times daily.
• Note color of sputum during the day (NOT IN THE MORNING). Yellow, green or brown indicates a bacterial infection, which will require an antibiotic.

3. Treatment:

• Rest. Go to bed if feverish.
• Drink liquids—aim for one 8-oz. glass every hour.
• Humidify air with cold vapor.
• Use postural drainage technique twice daily (see below).
• Take cough medicine, especially at night.
• Massage chest and back muscles to increase blood flow.
• Stop smoking (and never start again).

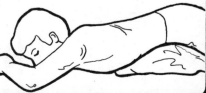

BURN WITH BLISTERS

Description: A blistering burn resulting from heat, chemicals or radiation.

What you need to know:

• Second-degree burns occur when tissue injury allows blood plasma to leak out of blood vessels into surrounding tissue and forms a blister.

• Burns are more serious for the young and old because they disturb fluid balance.

Get professional help if:

• Burn covers more than 10% of body surface.

• Areas of brown or blackened skin (third-degree burn) are evident.

• Under 14 or over 64 years old.

• Persistent pain is not relieved by aspirin.

Home Care:

Supplies: tape
gauze dressing
or cloth strips

burn ointment
or petroleum jelly
ice

1. Does burn cover more than 10% of body surface? If so, this causes shifts in body fluids, which may require hospitalization. Such extensive burns should *not* be covered with dressings or oil-based substances.

2. If less than 10% of body burned, apply cold water or ice to burn area (see p. 123). for *1 hour*, washing with mild soap.

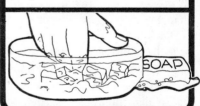

3. Apply oil-based substance (medicated ointment or sterile petroleum jelly). Cover with sterile gauze bandage or strips of clean cloth. Tape dressing loosely in place. Elevate burned area to help drainage. Keep it motionless to facilitate healing. Bed rest may be needed when feet or lower legs are burned.

4. Keep dressings on for 1 week unless they become soaked with plasma or develop an unpleasant odor. In that case, change them. To remove dressing, rinse with lots of cold water.

CHEST PAIN/HEART ATTACK

Description: Pain in chest that radiates into left arm, often with nausea, clammy skin, irregular heartbeat.

What you need to know:	*Get professional help if:*
• About 90% of suspected cases of chest pain are not due to heart attack but to a wide variety of musculo-skeletal, gastrointestinal, emotional and pulmonary causes. • The first few hours are most critical in dealing with heart attacks, yet the classic signs are present in only 60–70% of the cases. If the heart attack is real, you can tell with the Self-Test below.	• Your answers for the Self-Test below are *yes.* Immediately CALL THE RESCUE SQUAD and get to a hospital. (Transfer later on to a coronary unit may be needed.) • Your chest pain has persisted for 15 minutes.

Self-Test for Chest Pain

The following questions are designed to determine the odds that your chest pain is really a sign of a heart attack. "No" answers will indicate other causes of your chest pain. If you answer "yes" to most questions, CALL FOR HELP.

1. Place tip of index finger over center of chest pain; estimate distance (in inches) from centerline of chest. Is finger tip *2" or less* from line? (If yes, go to Step 2.)

2. Is the pain *above or even* with the nipple line? (If yes, go to Step 3.)

3. Is the pain *between* nipple and centerline? (If yes, go to Step 4.)

4. Is there pain on the *right side* of the chest? (If yes, go to Step 5.)

5. Can discomfort be described as a *dull pressure* or squeezing sensation under the necktie area? (If yes, go to Step 6.)

6. Is pain *continuous* (not coming and going)? (If yes, go to Step 7.)

7. Does discomfort last *at least* 5 to 10 minutes? (If yes, go to Step 8.)

8. Does pain *radiate* out to the arms, neck, jaws or any combination thereof? (If yes, go to Step 9.)

9. Is the discomfort *inside* of the arm? (If yes, go to Step 10.)
Note: To further evaluate arm discomfort, raise your arm over your head. If painful, stop. This type of pain is most likely caused by bursitis or shoulder arthritis.

10. Is there *sweating* with the pain? (If yes, go to Step 11.)

11. Is discomfort worse while *lying down?* (If yes, go to Step 12.)

12. If you've answered "yes" to most of the above questions, CALL FOR PROFESSIONAL HELP. It is quite likely that you need further study.

This test was originally designed as a telephone screening quiz by Glenn O. Turner, M.D.

Chest Pain Chart

The most common conditions that can cause chest pain are noted below, with a description of the characteristics of the pain and any associated symptoms.

	Heart Pain (Angina)	Gall Bladder Spasm	Stomach (Hiatal) Hernia	Anxiety
Pain Location	Chest midline; may spread across chest.	Upper abdomen; may spread to chest midline.	Upper abdomen and chest; often no symptoms.	Variable or over left chest.
Extent of Pain	Arms, neck, jaw; any combination of them.	Lower ribs to back, beneath right shoulder, left region and shoulder.	Arms, neck, jaw, or combinations of them.	Generally none.
Length of Pain	Usually 1-5 min.	Usually constant for hours; intermittent colic sometimes.	2 min. - 1 hour.	Less than 1 min. to a few hours.
Type of Pain	Heavy pressure or discomfort.	Severe, rapidly intensifying pain.	Dull discomfort.	Discomfort or sharp stabbing pain.
Related Symptoms	Indigestion.	Upper abdominal discomfort, nausea, vomiting, bloating, belching, dark urine.	Heartburn, hiccups, belching.	Jitters, worries, nervous stomach.
Causes	Exertion, emotion, foods, cold.	Large meals, fried foods.	Bending over, lying down, heavy meals.	Fatigue, emotion, stress.
Relief	Stop effort, take medicine.	Drink liquids, watch diet.	Drink liquids, sit or stand upright, take antacids.	Lie down, manage stress better, take medications.

Home Care:

Supplies: blood pressure unit   thermometer
stethoscope   watch with second hand

1. Symptoms:

Musculo-skeletal causes
- Chest wall aching worsened by deep breathing or twisting movement of upper body.
- Localized tenderness over ribs following history of fall or chest trauma.
- Neck pain worsened by movement of head and neck. May also produce aching in chest or upper arm.

Gastrointestinal causes
- Tenderness of abdomen at centerline (imaginary line from belly button to Adam's apple) under ribs, with related burning in stomach.
- Intermittent pain in upper abdomen on right, occasionally radiating to back under right shoulder blade (gall bladder problems).
- Burning pain at centerline, under ribs, that radiates to the jaws. Worsened by lying flat (esophagitis). Often occurs in obese people.

Emotional causes
- Chest pain associated with anxiety or stressful conditions.
- Chest pain related to hyper-ventilation (excessive rate and depth of respiration, causing abnormal loss of carbon dioxide from blood), due to emotional upset.

Pulmonary causes
- Chest pain in young adults or adults who have asthma or chronic obstructive pulmonary disease.
- Sudden shortness of breath, apprehension, sweating and faintness in people with history of phlebitis (inflammation of veins in legs) or calf pain, or while legs are immobilized for surgery or other reasons.

2. What to check:

- Take Self-Test (p. 140).
- Take blood pressure and record.
- Check pulse and record.
- Note breathing rate and record.
- Take temperature and record.

3. Treatment:

- If pain has persisted for more than 15 minutes, ask someone to take you to the nearest hospital. If no one can help you, call the rescue squad.
- Lie down and rest. Do not drive the car yourself!
- Tell the emergency room attendant you may be having a heart attack and insist on going to the coronary care unit — even if you only suspect a heart attack!

CHOKING

Description: Obstruction of the airway caused by object or food lodged in passage.

What you need to know:	Get professional help if:

What you need to know:

- Look for these 3 signals: bluish face and lips, complete collapse, and inability to speak.
- You can learn more about the Heimlich hug in CPR courses.

Get professional help if:

- Choking occurs. Have someone else CALL RESCUE SQUAD for assistance while you begin this procedure.

Home Care:

1. For standing patient, stand behind and wrap your arms around patient's waist. Make a fist, and use other hand to grab it. Place against patient's abdomen, slightly above navel and below rib cage. Press into abdomen with quick upward thrust. Repeat if necessary.

2. For patient lying down on back, kneel astride patient's hips, facing him. Put 1 hand on top of the other; apply heel of bottom hand on abdomen above navel and below rib cage. Press into abdomen with quick upward thrust.

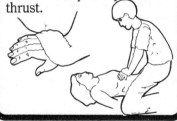

3. For sitting patient, stand behind patient's chair. Follow Step 1. For patient alone, apply force just below your abdomen by pressing into a table, chair or sink, or by using your own fist.

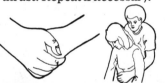

4. For child, turn child upside down over one arm in a jack-knife position. Apply blows to the back between shoulder blades.

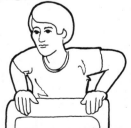

COMMON COLD

Description: A virus-caused inflammation of nasal and throat membranes; frequently involves ears and chest.

What you need to know:

- Colds last 3–7 days.
- Symptoms usually subside after third day.
- Antibiotics such as penicillin or tetracycline have no value in treating colds and may make them worse by creating resistant bacteria strains and/or diarrhea or stomach upset.

Get professional help if:

- Temperature over 101° several times in 1 day.
- Earache, sinus pain or chest pain develops.
- Coughing produces green or gray sputum.
- White or yellow spots on tonsils or throat.
- No improvement after 4 days.

Home Care:

Supplies: thermometer   hot salt water gargles   penlight
spoon handle as   nose drops   glasses of water
tongue depressor   aspirin   throat lozenges

1. Symptoms:

- bad breath
- breathing problems
- chills/fever
- congested or runny nose
- ear, neck, head aches
- postnasal drip, sneezing
- sore throat

2. What to check:

- Check temperature 3 times daily.
- Look down throat and record findings.
- Check number and location of enlarged lymph nodes.

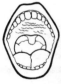

3. Treatment:

- Drink 8 oz. of water or juice each hour.
- Eat chicken soup—it actually has decongestant and curative properties!
- Gargle with hot salt water every 2 hours to relieve throat pain and clear mucus (see p. 122).

- Apply nose drops twice daily.
- Take aspirin for pain or fever.
- Use throat lozenges for sore throat.
- Wash hands and face frequently to prevent infecting others.
- Rest. Go to bed if fever exists.

CONVULSION

Description: Involuntary twitching and tremors of muscle groups followed by period of unconsciousness.

What you need to know:

- Convulsions are most common in children with high fevers.
- Unconsciousness may range from a few moments of confusion to deep sleep.
- Convulsions, in themselves, rarely cause death; main hazards are injuries to head during seizure.

Get professional help if:

- A convulsion of any kind occurs in adults or children. CALL RESCUE SQUAD for assistance and transportation.

Home Care:

Supplies: pen
paper
safety or straight pin

1. Symptoms:

- biting tongue
- blacking out
- breathing trouble
- chills/fever
- "funny feeling" before or after
- heart palpitations
- headache; stiff neck
- nausea, vomiting

2. What to check:

- During convulsion, check airway (open the airway if necessary—see p. 137). Only put fingers in mouth with extreme caution.
- Remove objects the person might hit.
- Gently restrain the person (no need to grasp tongue).

3. Treatment:

- DO NOT MOVE person unless necessary for safety. DO NOT put fingers in mouth.
- Loosen collar and tight clothing. Turn person on side.
- Check airway and skin color.
- Examine personal effects for medical card or ID tag showing history of epilepsy.

- Write down information gathered on paper, and pin to person or give to rescue squad.

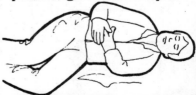

CUT/WOUND

Description: Any break in skin, such as an abrasion, laceration, puncture or cut.

What you need to know:

- When injury occurs, don't panic; this increases heart rate and speeds loss of blood. KEEP CALM.
- Over 50% of all cuts/wounds can be handled safely without professional help.

Get professional help if:

- Deep wound longer than 1".
- Bleeding, pain persists.
- Caused by human, animal bite.
- Last tetanus shot was 5 years ago (after a contaminated wound) or 10 years ago (after a clean wound).
- Wound is "dirty" (occurring outdoors or in farmyard).

Home Care:

Supplies: gauze dressings   antibacterial ointment
                    ice cubes   soap and water
                    plastic bag

1. If bleeding, apply *direct pressure* to wound with clean cloth. Continue pressure for 3 minutes.

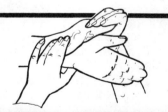

2. If bleeding is not profuse, apply ice in plastic bag to minimize swelling. Wash wound if dirty, making sure particles are flushed out.

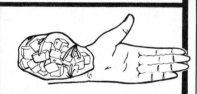

3. Apply antibacterial ointment. If necessary, use butterfly closures to pull edges together (see p. 125). Dress wound.

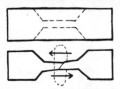

4. If cut is on finger or toe, tape to adjacent digit. If elsewhere, use tape or splint to keep injured area immobile. Change dressing daily.

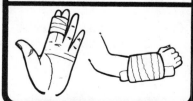

EARACHE

Description: An inflammation of the middle ear, usually caused by bacterial infection.

What you need to know:

- Otitis media is most common in children and adolescents but may be found in people of all ages.
- Ampicillin is often used as the antibiotic.
- Bacterial infections of middle ear in children under 3 years old may be painless (thus unnoticed).

Get professional help if:

- Patient is under 3 years old.
- Pain increases despite treatment.
- Dizziness develops.
- Temperature is over 102°.
- Ear drum ruptures. Look for reddish fluid draining from ear.
- Convulsive twitching of face muscles starts.

Home Care:

Supplies: otoscope
nose drops
Debrox ear drops
hot water bottle or heating pad

1. Symptoms:

- aching/pain/sound in ear
- chills/fever
- congestion, runny nose
- dizziness
- ear discharge
- fussing/tugging ear (child)
- headache
- hearing loss

2. What to check:

- Look at ear drum with otoscope. Gently pull ear upward as shown to straighten canal.

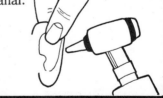

3. Treatment:

- Apply nose drops *immediately;* sniff 2–3 drops in nostril on same side as earache. Turn head with "bad ear" down after application.
- If ear drum appears black or brown, clean dark wax out using Debrox.

- Say "K–K–K" for 1 minute after dosing to draw the nose drops into the back of nose, near the eustachian tube.
- Apply heat to ear with hot compress (see p. 121).
- Rest; go to bed if there is fever.

FINGERNAIL/TIP INJURY

Description: Blow to fingertip causing intense pain, swelling, and black-and-blue fingernail.

What you need to know:

- Over 90% of fingertip injuries can be treated at home.
- When fingertip receives hard blow, the nail turns black and blue in several hours. Intense pain comes from accumulated blood trapped between nail and bone. Releasing the blood reduces the pain.

Get professional help if:

- Bony deformity suggests fracture or dislocation.
- Inability to straighten finger suggests damage to tendon.
- Drilling (below) impossible — patient uncooperative, tip badly swollen or patient alone.
- Pain persists after drilling.

Home Care:

Supplies: ice   Bandaid (gauze type)
                sharp blade or penknife
                cloth or gauze

1. Apply ice or cold water as soon as possible to reduce swelling (see p. 123).

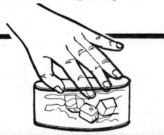

2. Have assistant hold finger or stabilize it yourself. Drill hole in nail using point of sharp blade. (Or use hot tip of paper clip.)

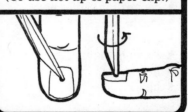

3. When hole is through nail, place tip of gauze or cloth into hole to absorb blood. Pain should be relieved immediately.

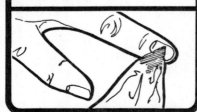

4. Cover hole with a gauze-type (not Telfa) bandage so blood continues to drain. Keep nail covered for a few days.

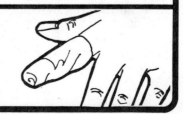

FOREIGN OBJECT IN EYE

Description: Foreign particles, chips or other materials lodged in sensitive eye tissue.

What you need to know:

- Do not rub or further irritate eye after injury.
- Normal tearing will occur immediately — tears may wash out the particle.

Get professional help if:

- Foreign object was impelled at high speed.
- History of previous injury with scarring of cornea.
- Foreign object cannot be removed in 2 or 3 attempts.
- Patient has only 1 good eye and foreign body is in that eye.

Home Care:

Supplies: penlight   matchstick
                 handkerchief
                 water to wash out eye

1. Wash out eye with cold water. Face assistant, looking in opposite direction while assistant locates object. Touch with corner of handkerchief.

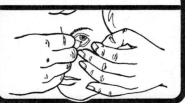

2. If object is beneath upper lid, have assistant grasp its lashes between thumb and index finger; while patient is looking *down,* pull upper lid over *lower* lid.

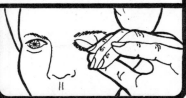

3. Another way to remove objects under upper lid is to "flip" the eyelid with a matchstick.

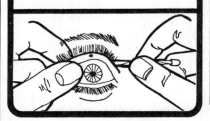

4. After object is removed, DO NOT RUB EYE; it will be sensitive for several hours. Reduce visual activities for 24 hours; avoid bright light or sunlight without sunglasses.

FOREIGN OBJECT IN LIMB

Description: Foreign objects such as splinters, thorns, fish hooks or glass slivers embedded in tissue.

What you need to know:

- Most objects close to skin surface are easily removed.

Get professional help if:

- Object is deeply imbedded.
- Affected area shows swelling or red streaks; OR lymph nodes are swollen 2–3 days after injury.
- Booster shot for tetanus is needed (should have booster every 10 years after third initial injection or after clean wound, and 5 years after contaminated wound).

Home Care:

Supplies: soap and water   Bandaid
                 ice
                 large sewing needle or tweezers

1. Before attempting extraction, scrub skin carefully with soap and water. Sterilize tweezers and needle over flame or in boiling water.

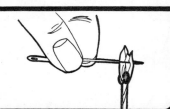

2. Locate object. Numb area with ice cube. With point of needle, slightly enlarge wound to make extraction easier.

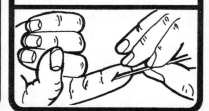

3. Flick out splinter or particle with needle or grasp it with tweezers. If object is fish hook, expose and clip barb as below.

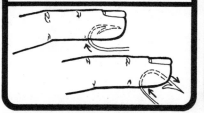

4. After extraction, cleanse again with soap and water. Cover with Bandaid. If finger or toe is affected, tape it to adjacent digit. Use splint to immobilize other areas (see p. 124). Soak puncture site in hot water for 20–30 minutes twice daily for 1 week. Change dressing daily for 1 week. (See p. 125.)

HIGH BLOOD PRESSURE

Description: Elevation of blood pressure above usually normal limits.

What you need to know:

• Hypertension has been called the "silent disease" because it may exist for years without apparent symptoms.

• Normal blood pressure is 130/80 or less. At 150/90, regardless of age, treatment is considered.

Get professional help if:

• Unexplained numbness of lips, face or arms occurs.

• Heart palpitations, skipped beats or shortness of breath occurs.

• Reaction to blood pressure medication is suspected, such as weakness, blurred vision, depression, fatigue, constipation, dizziness.

Home Care:

Supplies: blood pressure unit (electronic or aneroid) stethoscope

1. Symptoms:

• black-out spells; dizziness
• blurred or lost vision
• fatigue, depression
• headache
• insomnia; irritability
• numbness of lips, face, arms
• paralysis/weakness/twitching

2. What to check:

• Check blood pressure weekly.

• Check body weight and calculate ideal weight according to height. Female: 100 + 5 lbs. for each inch over 60 in. Male: 106 + 6 lbs. for each inch over 60 in.

3. Treatment:

• Lose weight if 20% over "ideal weight."

• Cut down salt in diet.

• Stop smoking.

• Avoid coffee, tea and cola drinks; caffeine elevates blood pressure.

• Maintain regular vigorous exercise for 20 minutes, 3 times a week.

• If on medication for hypertension, take as prescribed.

• Learn to control or cope with stress.

• Take regular vacations and use weekends wisely for rest and recreation.

INSECT BITE/STING

Description: Pain and reaction to venom that follows insect bite or sting of wasp, bee or hornet.

What you need to know:

• A few people (about 4%) experience a severe allergic reaction to stings. Left untreated, it can be fatal.

• Usually the pain and welt will subside in 3–4 hours.

• Keeping calm will keep the venom from spreading suddenly and triggering a reaction.

Get professional help if:

• Evidence of severe allergic reaction: swelling, itching eyes or lips; shortness of breath, wheezing; clammy, bluish skin; abdominal cramps, nausea.

• Family history of allergic reactions to stings.

• Known allergies.

• Multiple stings.

Home Care:

Supplies: Adolph's Meat Tenderizer   ice
aspirin   baking soda
clean cloth or gauze   household ammonia

1. In allergic reaction, stop spread of venom by firmly gripping area between site and heart. Get professional help.

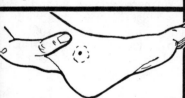

2. If no allergic reaction, remove stinger by scraping with fingernail or knife blade (don't use tweezers). Then wash area.

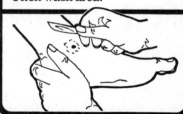

3. Put meat tenderizer on wet cloth or gauze. Place on sting for 20–30 minutes. Or apply ice or cold compresses (see p. 123).

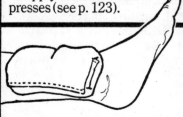

4. If itching or pain persists, apply baking soda/ammonia (½ cup soda with enough ammonia to make a paste) to skin. Take aspirin for pain. For next 2–3 days, try to avoid sweating, which may renew irritation.

NOSEBLEED

Description: Bleeding from nose caused by injury, common cold, allergies, dry climate or cracked, infected mucous surface.

What you need to know:

- The direct pressure method (below) will control 90% of bleeding from nose.
- No matter what the cause, blood from nose nearly always comes from front part of nose, not head or lungs.

Get professional help if:

- Bleeding is not controlled after repeating methods below 3 times.
- Difficulty in breathing.
- Taking anticoagulants.
- Nose has been broken.
- History of bleeding problems, blood disorders or high blood pressure.

Home Care:

Supplies: Vaseline

1. Squeeze nostrils firmly enough to stop bleeding without causing pain. (Gentle pressure may be applied to nose even if bones are broken.)

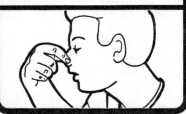

2. Lean trunk forward, still applying direct pressure. Do not lie down.

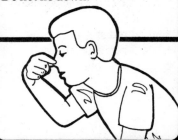

3. Continue applying pressure for full *5 minutes.* Relax. If bleeding recurs, continue pressure for 5 more minutes.

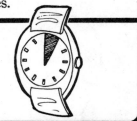

4. When bleeding is stopped, remain quiet for 2–3 hours. On third day after nosebleed, apply Vaseline inside nostrils twice daily.

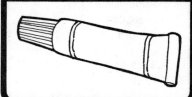

PINK EYE

Description: Inflammation of mucous covering of eye and eyelid, characterized by pink or bright red streaks.

What you need to know:

- Conjunctivitis is contagious.
- Serious eye conditions such as acute iritis, acute narrow-angle glaucoma and herpes simplex may cause similar symptoms.
- If pink eye occurs 6–8 hours after chipping paint or using grinding wheel, look for a tiny sliver of metal lodged in eye (see page 149).

Get professional help if:

- Distinct pain in eye itself or radiating to temple is felt.
- Vision changes or returning to well-lighted area after prolonged darkness (driving at night or after a movie) causes pain.
- Change in ability to see or in pupil size.
- No improvement after 24 hours.

Home Care:

Supplies: aspirin   eyedrops
white handkerchief   sunglasses

1. Symptoms:

- blurred or decreased vision
- headache
- itchy, red or watery eyes
- matter (mucus) in eyes
- swollen eyelids

2. What to check:

- Check for sandy, scratchy discomfort.
- Look for sticky mucus by touching it with corner of clean white handkerchief.
- Note any difference in size of pupils. A constricted pupil may indicate iritis (see above).

3. Treatment:

- Apply warm wet compresses to eyes 4 times a day for 10 minutes (see p. 121).
- Avoid wiping eyes.
- Take aspirin.
- Wear protective sunglasses.
- Get doctor's approval for use of prior prescription for eye drops.

- DO NOT USE EYE DROPS CONTAINING CORTISONE PREPARATIONS.

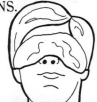

POISONING

Description: Life-threatening condition caused by ingestion of harmful solids, liquids or gases.

What you need to know:

- Children under 5 are especially susceptible to poisoning; they may taste medicines, cleaning products, chemicals or plants.
- Industrial or occupational exposure, accidental ingestion, suicide attempts and other factors cause adult poisoning.

Get professional help if:

- Poisoning of any kind occurs.
- CALL RESCUE SQUAD for assistance and transportation if victim is seriously ill.
- CALL POISON CONTROL CENTER for information and assistance.

Home Care:

Supplies: penlight
syrup of ipecac (for child)

1. Symptoms:

- abdominal pain; diarrhea
- black-out, unconsciousness
- blurred vision; convulsions
- choking, trouble breathing
- confusion, drowsiness
- coughing up blood; nausea
- dizziness, behavior change
- rash, burn

2. What to check:

- Check victim's breath for odors.
- Note significant objects near victim.
- Check lips and mouth for caustic burns.
- Shine penlight at pupil; if it doesn't constrict, suspect poisoning.

3. Treatment:

- CALL POISON CONTROL CENTER.
- Open windows and doors *quickly* if in closed room.
- Clear airway; do emergency breathing if necessary (see p. 137).
- If toxic substance is ingested by mouth and container is found, *administer antidote* according to label.
- Induce vomiting (EXCEPT for caustic lyes; or if victim is unconscious or having convulsions). Use finger in throat for adults, syrup of ipecac for children.

PSYCHIATRIC EMERGENCY

Description: Emotional crisis associated with alcohol or drug abuse, depression or acute psychiatric conditions.

What you need to know:

• Most common psychiatric emergency is "difficult drunk" or person experiencing hallucinations or delusions and violent paranoia. Both alcohol and mind-changing drugs can cause delirium.

• Other emergencies are severe depression, manic states and acute schizophrenic breakdown.

Get professional help if:

• Person seems dangerous (carrying firearms or weapons), unconscious or unresponsive to stimuli (questions, sounds). CALL RESCUE SQUAD for assistance and transportation.

Home Care:

Supplies: none

1. Symptoms:

• Because of unknown factors surrounding psychiatric emergencies, information about symptoms is not universally reliable.

• Alcohol/chemical abuse—alcoholics can become disoriented and visual or auditory hallucinations may accompany or precede DTs (delirium tremens).

• Drugs—psychedelic drugs may produce sensory aberrations and confusion.

• Depression—symptoms include insomnia, headache, fatigue, diminished sex drive, loss of appetite.

2. Treatment:

• Schizophrenia—contact a trained professional, as patient can be dangerous if armed with firearms or weapons.

• Violent behavior—a person who goes berserk may need to be restrained for safety's sake. A good rule of thumb is "4 for 1."

• Depression—if suicide is attempted or threatened, try to keep the person talking while awaiting aid.

• Lesser psychiatric emergencies—seek help from a qualified professional.

SCIATICA/BACK PAIN

Description: A common back disorder in which pain radiates down the back of the leg.

What you need to know:	*Get professional help if:*

What you need to know:

- When semicartilaginous "shock absorber" located between bony vertebrae deteriorates or is injured, pain may result.
- Inferior level of fitness or neglect of spinal flexibility exercises may lead to sciatica.

Get professional help if:

- Numbness in leg persists.
- History of repeated sciatica attacks.
- Pain remains after treatment plan.

Home Care:

Supplies: pillows   aspirin
             firm mattress
             kitchen-type chair

1. Take prompt preventive action. Change position; adjust car seat; avoid low chairs; be sure to lift properly.

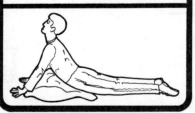

2. If pain or distress persists despite prompt protective action, intravertebral disc may have already protruded enough to irritate sciatic nerve.

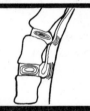

3. Perform hyperextension: lie face down with 2 pillows under chest. Or lean with hands against surface; bend back and head backward.

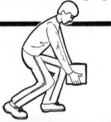

4. During the next 2–3 days: Do moderate work, but no lifting. Maintain proper sitting and standing posture. Do hyperextension exercise 3 times a day. Rest for 20 minutes each noon, lying flat on floor or firm mattress. Sit only on kitchen-type chairs. Take aspirin for pain.

SHOCK

Description: Life-threatening depression of vital body functions caused by injury, infection, heart attack, poisoning.

What you need to know:

• Degree of shock may be altered by age, body temperature, general health, reaction to stress or pain, handling of patient and treatment.

Get professional help if:

• Person goes into shock (see p. 126). CALL RESCUE SQUAD for assistance and transportation.

Home Care:

Supplies: blankets or heavy coats
blood pressure unit
watch with second hand

1. Symptoms:

• bluish skin
• chills, shaking, shivering
• dizziness, unconsciousness
• moist, clammy skin
• nausea, vomiting
• numbness, pain
• thirst
• trouble breathing

2. What to check:

• Check skin/mucous linings of mouth for color: pale or bluish?
• Check skin: is it moist?
• Check pulse at wrist or angle of jaw: is rate over 100/minute? weak or steady?
• Check blood pressure: less than 100/60?

3. Treatment:

• Clear airway.
• DO NOT MOVE patient unless necessary for safety.
• Loosen collar and tight clothing and turn patient on side.

• Cover patient lightly.
• Keep patient *lying down;* elevate legs 10–12".

SHOULDER OR ELBOW PAIN

Description: Soft-tissue injury to shoulder or elbow joint caused by overuse.

What you need to know:

- Rather than the specific sport or action, it is the *motion* involved with twisting or lifting that causes pain and limitations of joint.
- Cause may be improper conditioning or neglected warm-ups.

Get professional help if:

- Joint is swollen; it may require tapping and fluid drainage.
- Pain persists after 2–3 days of home treatment.
- History of previous attacks of bursitis or tendonitis.

Home Care:

Supplies: ColdHot Pack (3M)
aspirin
triangle sling

1. Symptoms:

- ache/pain in shoulder, elbow
- limited motion of joint
- sleep loss due to pain
- stiffness
- swelling in joint

2. What to check:

- Check joint for swelling (which may be extensive) and fluid accumulation.
- Note events leading to attack and motions that aggravate condition.

3. Treatment:

Immediate treatment plan:
- Apply cold for first 24 hours, 3 times a day for 10–15 minutes (see p. 123).
- Apply heat for next 48 hours, 3 times a day for 10–15 minutes (see p. 121).
- Take aspirin for pain.
- Use triangle sling.

Follow-up treatment plan:
- Gently massage muscles.

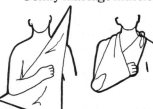

SINUS INFECTION

Description: Inflammation and infection of sinus cavities in cheekbones and forehead.

What you need to know:

- Maxillary (cheekbone) sinusitis is most common form of sinus infection.
- About 50% of sinus infections are caused by viruses; other 50% are bacterial and are helped by antibiotics.

Get professional help if:

- Temperature over 101° several times a day.
- Bleeding from nose.
- Blurring or change in vision.
- Increased thick nasal discharge.
- Increased swelling of forehead, eye area, sides of nose, cheeks.

Home Care:

Supplies: thermometer   glasses of water
                     nose drops
                     hot salt water gargles

1. Symptoms:

- bad breath
- bloody nose
- blurred vision, headache
- chills/fever
- postnasal drip
- runny or congested nose
- tenderness over forehead, cheek

2. What to check:

- Note temperature 3 times daily.
- Is headache worse when bending over to touch toes?
- Are forehead and cheekbones tender to touch?
- Gently blow nose and examine discharge. Yellow or streaked with blood?

3. Treatment:

- At first sign of distress, use alternating hot and cold compresses over face twice daily. Apply each for 5–10 minutes (see pp. 121–123).
- Apply nose drops after using compresses. Sniff 2–3 drops into each nostril. Say "K–K–K" for 1 minute.

- Gargle to clear out mucus (see p. 122).
- Increase fluid intake.
- Stop smoking.
- Rest; go to bed if feverish.

SORE THROAT

Description: Inflammation of throat caused by viral or bacterial infection.

What you need to know:

- Over 80% of sore throats are caused by viruses and are not helped by antibiotics.
- Main complication is "strep" infection caused by Group A, beta-hemolytic streptococcus bacteria. It can only be determined by throat culture.

Get professional help if:

- Sore throat persists for 5 days.
- Fever over 101° several times a day.
- Rash develops.
- History of rheumatic fever, kidney disease or frequent strep infection.

Home Care:

Supplies:

thermometer	penlight	glasses of water
spoon handle as	hot salt water	aspirin
tongue depressor	hot liquids	lozenges

1. Symptoms:

- bad breath
- chills/fever
- head, neck aches
- hoarseness
- lymph nodes in neck enlarged or tender
- runny or congested nose
- sore throat

2. What to check:

- Check temperature 3 times daily and record.
- Check throat color.
- Count swollen lymph nodes of neck; note location.

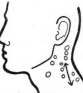

3. Treatment:

- Gargle with hot salt water every 2 hours to relieve pain and clear mucus (see p. 122).
- Take frequent sips of hot liquids such as lemonade or weak tea.
- Drink an 8-oz. glass of water or juice each hour to replace lost fluids.
- Take aspirin for pain or fever.
- Use throat lozenges to soothe rawness.
- Wash hands and face frequently to limit spread of infection.
- Stop smoking (and don't start again).
- Rest; go to bed if fever exists.

SPRAINED ANKLE

Description: Damage to ligaments or joint capsule of ankle following a twisting fall.

What you need to know:	*Get professional help if:*
• Sprained ankles tend to be underdiagnosed and undertreated, which can lead to lifelong disability—limping, unstable ankle; swollen ankle; foot pain; or difficulty on rough terrain. • Severity of sprain often has no relation to severity of complications.	• Ankle is twisted. Because of difficulties in evaluating ankle injuries, most sprains should be seen by physician.

Home Care:

Supplies: ice   crutches
                    pillows
                    elastic bandage

1. Follow these steps as needed, with professional's advice. Apply ice or cold compress (see p. 123) for 1 hour.

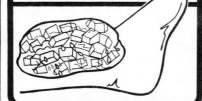

2. Immobilize ankle by elevating on 2–3 pillows for 24 hours. Wrap firmly with elastic bandage to control swelling (see p. 125).

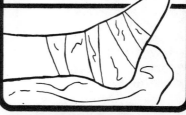

3. There are 2 methods of sprain treatment; physician will choose best method. *Non-weight-bearing*—wrap in elastic bandage, use crutches and stay off foot for 1 week (mild sprain) or 2 weeks (severe sprain). *Early weight-bearing*—apply cast or basketweave tape splint (see p. 124). Use crutches for 3 weeks.

4. If elastic bandage is used, remove twice a day for hot soak and ankle massage. Later wear ankle-supporting boots.

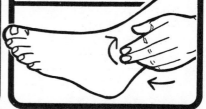

STOMACH FLU

Description: Disorder of digestive system with nausea, vomiting, diarrhea.

What you need to know:

• About 90% of gastroenteritis cases are caused by viruses and run their course in 24–48 hours.

• Diarrhea may be PROTEC-TIVE, as the body speeds offending particles through digestive tract. So don't take antidiarrheal medication during first 6–8 hours.

Get professional help if:

• More than 8 stools or bouts of diarrhea occur per day.

• Temperature over 101° several times a day.

• Black or bloody stools, vomit.

• Infant, young child, diabetic, chronically ill, or elderly.

• No improvement after 24 hours of home treatment.

Home Care:

Supplies: thermometer   clear liquids (tea, broth)
ice chips
soft foods

1. Symptoms:

• abdominal pain, stomachache
• chills/fever
• diarrhea
• dry mouth
• headache
• muscle aches
• nausea, vomiting

2. What to check:

• Note temperature 3 times daily.
• Note location and pattern of pain if present (see p. 130).
• Record number and kind of stools.
• Is anyone who ate the same meal sick? Has victim returned from a foreign area?

3. Treatment:

• Rest in bed until nausea, vomiting, diarrhea and fever are gone.

• Keep flat. An upright position increases amount of fluid lost during bouts of diarrhea.

Food and liquid intake:

• Day 1—ice chips only, until vomiting subsides.

• Day 2—clear liquids, sweetened tea, ginger ale or broth.

• Day 3—soft foods, custard, baked potato, cooked cereal, pudding, Jello.

• For next 5 days—avoid alcohol, spicy foods and fruits; they may bring back symptoms.

STROKE

Description: Brain injury that results from spontaneous rupture of a blood vessel or formation of clot.

What you need to know:

• A stroke may be *major* (a cardiovascular accident, or CVA, with paralysis or weakness along one side of body) or *minor* (a transient ischemic attack, or TIA—see symptoms listed below). TIA tells you too little blood is reaching the brain and warns you that CVA could follow within five years.

Get professional help if:

• A stroke of any kind occurs. CALL RESCUE SQUAD for assistance and transportation if *major stroke.*

Home Care:

Supplies: blood pressure unit
watch with second hand

1. Symptoms:

• black-out, unconsciousness
• confusion, drowsiness
• difficulty breathing, swallowing, speaking
• clumsiness
• personality change
• numbness of hand, foot
• paralysis/twitching/ weakness

2. What to check:

• Check mental awareness: ask name, time of day, place.
• Ask person to repeat short sentence to test speech.
• Ask person to rise and walk a few steps with your assistance: dizzy? staggering gait?
• Check blood pressure and pulse (see pp. 106–107).

3. Treatment:

If major stroke:
• Check airway; clear of vomit, food, dentures.
• DO NOT MOVE victim unless necessary for safety.
• Loosen collar or tight clothing; turn victim on side.

If minor stroke:
• Have person evaluated by physician as soon as possible.

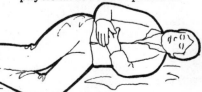

UNCONSCIOUSNESS

Description: A coma that results from drug or alcohol intoxication, head injury or illness such as diabetes.

What you need to know:	*Get professional help if:*

What you need to know:

- Most common cause is alcohol intoxication or sleeping pill overdose. Second most common is head injury.
- Other causes are stroke, diabetic coma, insulin reaction, overdose of legal or illegal drug, carbon monoxide poisoning, inhalation of industrial gas.

Get professional help if:

- Unconsciousness occurs. CALL RESCUE SQUAD for assistance and transportation.

Home Care:

Supplies: pen
safety or straight pin
paper

1. Check airway; do emergency breathing if necessary (see p. 137). Clear out food, vomit, mucus, dentures.

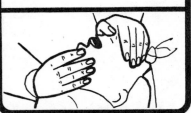

2. Turn victim to side. Note color of skin and lips.

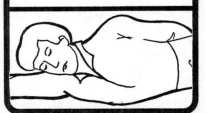

3. Check personal effects for medical card or "Medic-Alert" ID tag for important information. Look for a suicide note.

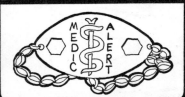

4. Write gathered information (medical data, next of kin, doctor's name) on paper, and pin to victim or give to rescue squad.

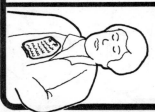

WRIST INJURY

Description: A sprain or break that occurs when wrist is bent (usually backward) beyond normal range.

What you need to know:	*Get professional help if:*

- The wrist is broken more often than any other bone; true sprains are rare.
- Fractures of the wrist may involve the 2 bones of the forearm (ulna and radius) or the 8 small carpal bones of hand and wrist.

- Wrist injury occurs. It is important to x-ray any wrist injury to determine whether a break requires casting or other treatment. Neglect of even a hairline fracture can lead to complications in the future.
- Pain or swelling is notable or bluish discoloration visible.

Home Care:

Supplies: ice
              elastic bandage
              magazine/newspaper   blanket or pillow

1. (Follow these steps before getting professional help.) To prevent shock (see p. 158), if person feels faint, lie flat on back; elevate forearm.

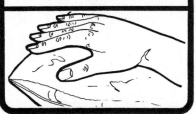

2. Apply cold or ice pack or use cold wet compresses for at least 30 minutes to minimize swelling (see p. 123).

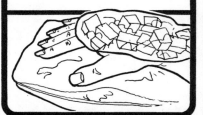

3. Splint arm and wrist with magazine/newspaper and elastic bandage. Support arm in sling (see p. 124).

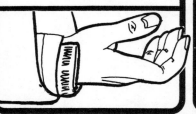

4. Check fingertips of injured arm repeatedly for swelling and bluish discoloration. If this occurs, loosen ties of splint or elastic bandage.

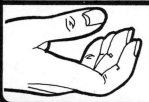

INDEX

Free Stuff!

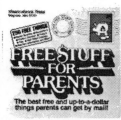

Free Stuff For Parents
Over 250 of the best free and up-to-a-dollar booklets and samples parents can get by mail: • *sample teether, baby spoon, safety latch and drinking cup* • *booklets on pregnancy, childbirth, child care, nutrition, health, safety, first aid, reading, day care* • *sample copies of parenting newsletters and magazines and mail order catalogs.* **Only $3.75 ppd.**

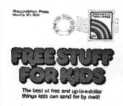

Free Stuff For Kids
Over 250 of the best free and up-to-a-dollar things kids can get by mail: • *badges & buttons* • *games, kits & puzzles* • *coins, bills & stamps* • *bumper stickers & decals* • *coloring & comic books* • *posters & maps* • *seeds & rocks.* FREE STUFF FOR KIDS is America's #1 best-selling book for children! **Only $3.75 ppd.**

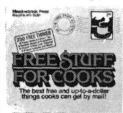

Free Stuff For Cooks
Over 250 of the best free and up-to-a-dollar booklets and samples cooks can get by mail: • *cookbooks with more than 3,700 recipes for cooking with almonds, fish, wine, eggs, in microwave ovens, clay pots and more* • *money-saving shopping guides and nutrition information* • *sample popcorn ball maker, herb seeds, spices* • *sample food and couponing newsletters.* **Only $3.75 ppd.**

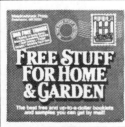

Free Stuff For Home & Garden
Over 350 of the best free and up-to-a-dollar booklets, catalogs and products the home handyman and gardener can get by mail: • *free plans for a new home or addition* • *22 ways to save energy heating and cooling a home* • *furniture-by-mail* • *sample seeds and plants* • *tips on landscaping and vegetable gardening* • *weatherproofing, insulating, and painting guides.* **Only $3.75 ppd.**

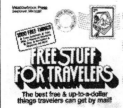

Free Stuff For Travelers
Over 1000 free and up-to-a-dollar things travelers can get by mail: • *camping information* • *colorful travel posters* • *festivals and free attractions* • *canoe trips and cruises* • *hotel and motel directories* • *state and national park information* • *beaches and resorts* • *skiing and sailing vacations* • *travel and safety tips* • *maps and guidebooks for thousands of destinations!* **Only $3.75 ppd.**

Meadowbrook's Tips

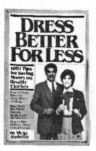

Dress Better For Less
by Vicki Audette
When, where and how to find bargains on new and used clothing for men, women and children. Get the clothes you really want — for much less than you ever thought possible! • *finding blue chip clothes in schlock shops* • *strategic shopping tips for finding bargains in 20 different kinds of retail outlets* • *directory of national bargain chains* • *shrewd tips for updating and repairing clothes* • *scouting designer fashions at discount houses.* **Only $5.75 ppd.**

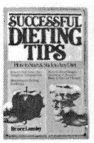

Successful Dieting Tips
Compiled by Bruce Lansky
The reason most diets don't work is that dieter's can't stick to them. SUCCESSFUL DIETING TIPS contains over 1,000 proven ideas to help dieters start and stick to any diet, such as how to: • *select the diet that's best for you* • *overcome toughest diet temptations of favorite foods, holidays, and eating out* • *avoid binges and bounce back when you can't resist* • *maintain an ideal weight.* **Only $5.75 ppd.**

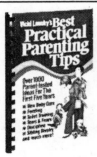

Best Practical Parenting Tips
by Vicki Lansky
Over 1,000 parent-tested ideas for baby and child care that you won't find in Dr. Spock's books. Vicki's newest bestseller is the most helpful collection of new, down-to-earth ideas from new parents ever published. Practical ideas for saving time, trouble and money on such topics as: • *new baby care* • *car travel* • *toilet training* • *dressing kids for less* • *discipline* • *self-esteem.* **Only $5.75 ppd.**

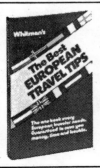

The Best European Travel Tips
by John Whitman
Here's what the other travel guides don't tell about Europe. Whitman's indispensable, easy-to-read tips tell how to avoid tourist traps, rip offs and snafus . . . and how to: • *avoid getting ripped-off on currency exchanges* • *get low-cost airfares, tours, hotel rates* • *get your travel documents quickly* • *get through customs quickly* • *how to beat no-vacancy at a hotel* • *how to keep your fanny from being pinched in Italy.* **Only $5.75 ppd.**

Free Things To Do And See

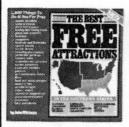

The Best Free Attractions South

From North Carolina to Texas, it's a land swarming with surprises – and over 1,500 of them free:

- *alligator and turtle stalking*
- *cow chip tosses & mule races*
- *free watermelon, bluegrass & barbeque!*

$4.75 ppd.

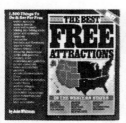

The Best Free Attractions West

"Just passin' through" from California to Montana? Here's over 1,500 free and exciting attractions for the asking:

- *belching volcanoes & miniature forests*
- *gold panning & quarter horse racing*
- *vineyard tours with free wine samples*

$4.75 ppd.

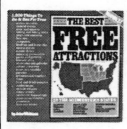

The Best Free Attractions Midwest

From Kentucky to North Dakota, the Midwest is chock-full of free things:

- *camel rides and shark feedings*
- *stagecoaches and magic tricks*
- *hobo conventions – and free Mulligan stew!*

$4.75 ppd.

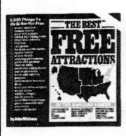

The Best Free Attractions East

Over 1,500 irresistible attractions – all free – from West Virginia to Maine:

- *a witchtrial courthouse – with evidence*
- *aviaries where you are caged*
- *the "gentle giants" – and free beer!*

$4.75 ppd.

Order Form

BOOKS (Prices include postage and handling.)

_____	BEST EUROPEAN TRAVEL TIPS	$5.75 ppd.
_____	BEST FREE ATTRACTIONS (EAST)	$4.75 ppd.
_____	BEST FREE ATTRACTIONS (MIDWEST)	$4.75 ppd.
_____	BEST FREE ATTRACTIONS (SOUTH)	$4.75 ppd.
_____	BEST FREE ATTRACTIONS (WEST)	$4.75 ppd.
_____	SUCCESSFUL DIETING TIPS	$5.75 ppd.
_____	DRESS BETTER FOR LESS	$5.75 ppd.
_____	FREE STUFF FOR COOKS	$3.75 ppd.
_____	FREE STUFF FOR HOME & GARDEN	$3.75 ppd.
_____	FREE STUFF FOR KIDS	$3.75 ppd.
_____	FREE STUFF FOR PARENTS	$3.75 ppd.
_____	FREE STUFF FOR TRAVELERS	$3.75 ppd.
_____	BEST PRACTICAL PARENTING TIPS	$5.75 ppd.
_____	FAMILY DOCTOR'S HEALTH TIPS	$5.75 ppd.

Name: _____

Address: _____

_____Zip _____

If ordering more than 6 books, please write to us for quantity discount rates.

$ Total enclosed _____

Make checks payable to:
Meadowbrook Press, Dept. **FDHT–DM**
I bought my book at ☐ bookstore ☐ other retail store ☐ my bookclub